Foreword

Pocket Tutor Ophthalmology continues the tradition of ophthalmology teaching in Edinburgh, established in 1883 when Douglas Argyll Robertson was appointed the first lecturer in diseases of the eye at the university.

For doctors not in the specialty, ophthalmology too often appears a mysterious subject with many acronyms, unpronounceable terms, and innumerable syndromes. In reality, and as this book emphasises, ophthalmology has the advantages that the eye is (mostly) visible and the diseases that affect it can be diagnosed logically, if an ordered approach to history taking and examination is adopted. For instance, patients with a vague complaint of visual blurring may harbour a potentially blinding condition that may be missed if the simple tests of pupillary function and visual field examination are omitted. For those in hospital practice, the importance of eye examination in relation to extraocular disease cannot be overemphasised. For example, a young patient with a headache may be harbouring a brain tumour, with the only sign being papilloedema seen on fundoscopy.

I confidently recommend *Pocket Tutor Ophthalmology* as an easily accessible guide to diagnosis and management for clinical students, trainee ophthalmologists, emergency doctors, general practitioners and anyone involved in the management of patients suffering from diseases of the central nervous system.

James F Cullen FRCS FRCSEd
Former Consultant Ophthalmologist, Edinburgh

Ophthalmology

Shyamanga Borooah BSc(Hons) MBBS MRCP(UK)
MRCSEd FRCOphth
Wellcome Trust Clinical Research Training Fellow
Scottish Translational Medicine and Therapeutics
Initiative
Honorary Registrar
Princess Alexandra Eye Pavilion
Edinburgh, UK

Mark Wright MBChB (Aberdeen) FRCSEd
Consultant Ophthalmologist
Princess Alexandra Eye Pavilion
Edinburgh, UK

Baljean Dhillon BMedSci (Hons) BM BS (Nottingham)
FRCSEd FRCPS(Glasg) FRCOphth
Honorary Professor of Ophthalmology
University of Edinburgh
SBE Visual Impairment Studies
Heriot-Watt University
Consultant Ophthalmologist
Princess Alexandra Eye Pavilion
Edinburgh, UK

JP
medical
publishers

© 2012 JP Medical Ltd.

Published by JP Medical Ltd, 83 Victoria Street, London, SW1H 0HW, UK

Tel: +44 (0)20 3170 8910 Fax: +44 (0)20 3008 6180

Email: info@jpmedpub.com Web: www.jpmedpub.com

ISBN: 978-1-907816-21-5

British Library Cataloguing in Publication Data
A catalogue record for this book is available from the British Library

Library of Congress Cataloging in Publication Data
A catalog record for this book is available from the Library of Congress

JP Medical Ltd is a subsidiary of Jaypee Brothers Medical Publishers (P) Ltd, New Delhi, India (www.jaypeebrothers.com).

Publisher:	Richard Furn
Development Editor:	Paul Mayhew
Editorial Assistant:	Katrina Rimmer
Design:	Designers Collective Ltd
Index:	Jill Dormon

Typeset, printed and bound in India.

Ophthalmology

pocket tutor

Preface

Eye diseases are amongst the most common conditions seen in hospital, contributing to approximately ten percent of all outpatient appointments. The majority of these eye conditions are often easily treatable once they have been diagnosed. In addition, a large number of systemic diseases have ocular manifestations.

Correct diagnosis and management can mean sight is saved, or even restored. Consequently, a sound understanding of the eye and its surrounding structures in health and disease is widely relevant in medicine. *Pocket Tutor Ophthalmology* aims to provide a concise and accessible reference to aid understanding and diagnosis of common ophthalmological diseases.

Ophthalmology is often perceived as being difficult to access due to not only the specialised nature of the eye itself, but also the specialist terminology and equipment. This book helps simplify the approach to ocular examination by providing a sound platform of relevant anatomy and physiology. Chapter 2 takes the reader through the important examination techniques and investigations to assist diagnosis. Chapter 3 contains a series of algorithms, developed specifically for this book, which help make clinical diagnosis easier.

The clinical chapters are divided on an anatomical basis and although not exhaustive cover the most common conditions. Each chapter starts with a series of clinical scenarios that provide examples of how these conditions present in the clinical setting. The wonderful thing about ophthalmology is that most conditions can be diagnosed visually so the chapters contain many high-quality colour photographs of pathology.

This book has been written for for medical students, trainees, primary care practitioners and optometrists, to assist in the diagnosis of eye disease. The handy pocket size ensures portability and ease of use. We have made every effort to make *Pocket Tutor Ophthalmology* simple, clear and up-to-date and hope you will find it both enjoyable to read and clinically useful.

Shyamanga Borooah
Mark Wright
Baljean Dhillon
January 2012

Contents

Acknowledgements

We thank the following authors for their kind permission to reproduce figures from their books, published by Jaypee Brothers Medical Publishers (P) Ltd:

Agarwal S, Apple DJ, Agarwal A, Buratto L, Alió JL, Pandey SK, Agarwal A. Textbook of Ophthalmology. New Delhi: Jaypee Brothers Medical Publishers, 2002. Figures 1.16, 1.17.

Basak SK. Atlas on Clinical Ophthalmology. New Delhi: Jaypee Brothers Medical Publishers, 2006. Figures 2.9, 6.5, 7.1–7.6, 8.1–8.3, 10.2–10.4, 11.2, 11.10, 11.14, 12.12, 12.13, 12.14, 12.17, 13.3.

Bijlani RL. Understanding Medical Physiology: A Textbook for Medical Students (3rd Edition). New Delhi: Jaypee Brothers Medical Publishers, 2004. Figure 12.1.

Datta H. Strabismus. New Delhi: Jaypee Brothers Medical Publishers, 2004. Figure 1.2.

Garg A, Rosen E, Crouch ER, Oleszczynska-Prost E. Instant Clinical Diagnosis in Ophthalmology strabismus. New Delhi: Jaypee Brothers Medical Publishers, 2009. Figures 13.5, 13.7, 13.9.

Garg A, Rosen E, Melamed S, Dada T, Khalil AK. Instant Clinical Diagnosis in Glaucoma. New Delhi: Jaypee Brothers Medical Publishers, 2009. Figures 12.3, 12.9.

Garg A, Fry LL, Tabin G, Gutiérrez-Carmona FJ, Pandey SK. Clinical Practice in Small Incision Cataract Surgery (Phaco Manual). New Delhi: Jaypee Brothers Medical Publishers, 2004. Figure 1.18.

Garg A, Mortensen J, Marchini G. Mastering the Techniques of Glaucoma Diagnosis and Management. New Delhi: Jaypee Brothers Medical Publishers, 2006. Figure 12.10.

Garg A, Rosen E, Lee SH, Crouch ER, Oleszczynska-Prost E, Trivedi RH. Instant Clinical Diagnosis in Ophthalmology Pediatric

Ophthalmology. New Delhi: Jaypee Brothers Medical Publishers, 2009. Figures 14.1, 14.2.

Garg A, Rosen E, Mortensen J, El Toukhy E, Dhaliwal RS. Instant Clinical Diagnosis in Ophthalmology: Oculoplasty & Reconstructive Surgery. New Delhi: Jaypee Brothers Medical Publishers, 2008. Figures 6.3, 6.8b.

Garg A, Rosen E, Pérez-Arteaga A, Goyal JL. Instant Clinical Diagnosis in Ophthalmology: Neuro-ophthalmology. New Delhi: Jaypee Brothers Medical Publishers, 2009. Figure 12.4.

Garg A, Rosen E, Pérez-Arteaga A, Sharma A. Instant Clinical Diagnosis in Ophthalmology: Anterior Segment Diseases. New Delhi: Jaypee Brothers Medical Publishers, 2009. Figures 1.4, 15.1.

Garg A, Sheppard JD, Donnenfeld ED, Friedlaender M. Clinical Applications of Antibiotics & Anti-inflammatory Drugs in Ophthalmology. New Delhi: Jaypee Brothers Medical Publishers, 2007. Figure 6.6.

Garg A, Sheppard JD, Donnenfeld ED, Meyer D, Mehta CK. Clinical Diagnosis and Management of Dry Eye and Ocular Surface Disorders (Xero-Dacryology). New Delhi: Jaypee Brothers Medical Publishers, 2006. Figure 2.8.

Gupta AK, Choudhry RM, Tandon C. Step by Step Visual Field Examination. New Delhi: Jaypee Brothers Medical Publishers, 2007. Figure 12.8.

Gupta AK, Mazumdar S, Choudhry S. Practical Approach to Ophthalmoscopic Retinal Diagnosis. New Delhi: Jaypee Brothers Medical Publishers, 2010. Figure 1.19.

Mukherjee PK. Essentials of Neuro-Opthalmology. New Delhi: Jaypee Brothers Medical Publishers, 2010. Figures 1.3, 1.7.

Nema HV, Nema N. Textbook of Ophthalmology. New Delhi: Jaypee Brothers Medical Publishers, 2008. Figures 1.6, 1.8, 1.9, 1.11, 1.12, 4.1 –4.3, 6.1, 6.2, 6.4, 12.5, 12.7b, 12.11, 12.18.

Pandey SK. Dry Eye & Ocular Surface Disorders. New Delhi: Jaypee Brothers Medical Publishers, 2006. Figure 1.15.

Rani PK, Lingam G, Sharma T. The Sankara Nethralaya Atlas of Retinal Diseases. New Delhi: Jaypee Brothers Medical Publishers, 2008. Figure 1.5.

Saxena S. Clinical Practice in Ophthalmology. New Delhi: Jaypee Brothers Medical Publishers, 2003. Figure 1.14.

Singh I. Textbook of Human Histology. New Delhi: Jaypee Brothers Medical Publishers, 2007. Figures 1.10a, 1.10b, 1.20.

Singh I. Textbook of Human Osteology. New Delhi: Jaypee Brothers Medical Publishers, 2009. Figure 1.1.

Subrahmanyam M. Surgical Atlas of Orbital Diseases. New Delhi: Jaypee Brothers Medical Publishers, 2009. Figures 15.2, 15.3.

First principles

1.1 Anatomy

A basic knowledge of structure and function is necessary to understand how symptoms and signs relate to disease manifestations. From the front to the back of the eyeball, the structures are:

- the **cornea**, which is clear
- the **anterior chamber,** a clear fluid-filled region
- the **iris**, which is coloured and has a small aperture called the **pupil**, through which light passes
- the **lens**, a crystalline structure
- the **vitreous cavity**, a jelly-like cavity posterior to the lens
- the **retina**, a delicate neurovascular lattice at the back of the interior of the globe.

Beyond the clear cornea the exterior of the eyeball is composed of a robust collagenous structure known as the **sclera**. The globe sits within a bony orbit (**Figure 1.1**) with a periocular soft-tissue support. The eye rotates within the orbit by the action of the six **extraocular muscles** (**Figure 1.2**). Anteriorly the globe is protected by the eyelids. Posteriorly, the optic nerve, the main neural output of the eye, travels from the globe towards the brain, exiting the orbit via a small hole in the skull known as the **optic canal**, before decussating at the **optic chiasm** above the pituitary gland (**Figure 1.3**).

Clinical insight

Failure of fusion of the optic vesicle during embryonic development leads to a **coloboma**. Colobomas are seen as incomplete formations of the iris anteriorly and of the sclera, choroid and retina posteriorly along the line of the optic fissure (**Figure 1.5**).

Embryology

The eye forms from the **optic vesicle**, an outpouching from the primitive forebrain which invaginates to form a cup-like structure. It also folds along the optic fissure, the edges of which fuse inferonasally (**Figure 1.4**).

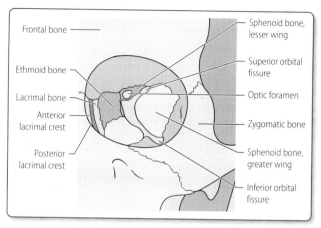

Figure 1.1 The skull and right orbit.

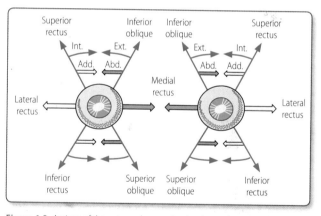

Figure 1.2 Actions of the extraocular muscles. Int., internal rotation; Ext., external rotation; Add., adduction; Abd., abduction.

Conjunctiva

The inner eyelid and ocular surface are covered in a stratified columnar epithelium called the **conjunctiva**. The **tarsal conjunctiva** on the inner aspect of the eyelids (**Figure 1.6**) is

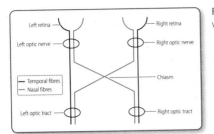

Figure 1.3 The anterior visual pathway.

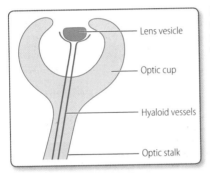

Figure 1.4 Invagination of the optic vesicle to form the optic cup and the choroidal fissure.

continuous with the **bulbar conjunctiva**, which covers the globe. The fornices, where the bulbar and tarsal conjunctiva join, are visible by retracting the lid and asking the patient to look in the opposite direction.

Cornea and sclera

The **cornea (Figure 1.7)** is a transparent, convex 'window' at the front of the eye that consists of five layers. It is composed of collagen fibrils that are aligned in such a way as to allow light to pass easily.

The cornea is one of the most highly innervated parts of the body with a subepithelial plexus of nerves. Any break in the contiguity of the corneal epithelium results in pain/irritation through activation of the trigeminal nerve and reflex lacrimation through activation of the facial nerve (**Figure 1.8**). This system has evolved in order to keep the cornea clear and free of foreign bodies.

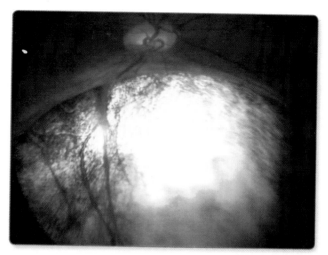

Figure 1.5 Coloboma of the posterior choroid.

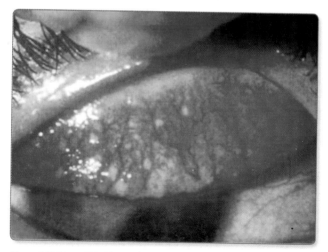

Figure 1.6 Everted lid with vernal conjunctivitis of the tarsal conjunctiva.

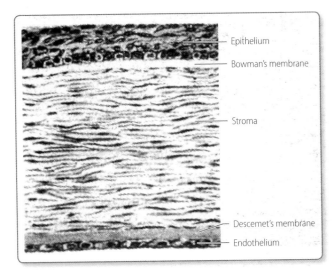

Figure 1.7 Corneal histology.

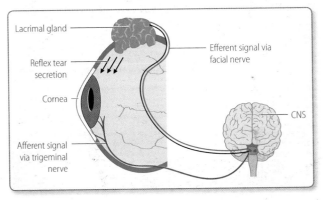

Figure 1.8 The reflex lacrimation loop. CNS, central nervous system.

The circumference of the round cornea is known as the **limbus**. Corneal stem cells are found at the limbus; these help to replace lost or damaged epithelial cells (**Figure 1.9**).

The **sclera** is continuous with the cornea at the limbus. It is visible through the transparent conjunctival mucosa as the white of the eye. It consists of a dense non-transparent arrangement of collagen. Attached to it are the extraocular muscles and periocular soft tissue.

Pupil

The **pupil** is the central aperture of the iris. Dilation of the pupil occurs via sympathetic signals to the radially arranged dilator pupillae muscles; constriction of the pupil occurs via parasympathetic signals to the circumferentially arranged constrictor pupillae muscle (**Figure 1.10**).

Lens

The crystalline **lens** (**Figure 1.11**) is composed of a multi-layered and interdigitating arrangement of lens fibrils that consist of crystalline proteins. These are laid down in chronological order of development such that the foetal nucleus is at the core of the lens and all the fibres are added to the outer layers, much like the rings of tissue in a tree trunk. There is a dense nuclear region surrounded by a softer cortex region, both of which are encapsulated by an elastic outer capsule to which lens **zonules**, fibres from the ciliary body controlling lens shape, are attached.

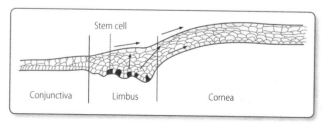

Figure 1.9 The migration of limbal stem cells to repair an abrasion.

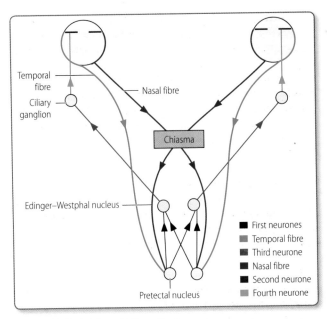

Figure 1.10 The pupil constriction pathway.

Temporal fibre
Ciliary ganglion
Nasal fibre
Chiasma
Edinger–Westphal nucleus
Pretectal nucleus

■ First neurones
■ Temporal fibre
■ Third neurone
■ Nasal fibre
■ Second neurone
■ Fourth neurone

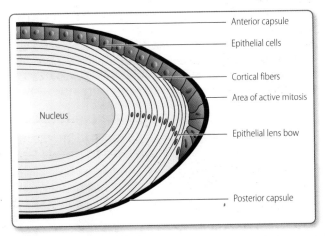

Figure 1.11 The structure of the lens.

Anterior capsule
Epithelial cells
Cortical fibers
Area of active mitosis
Epithelial lens bow
Posterior capsule
Nucleus

Vitreous humour

Behind the lens and filling most of the eyeball volume is the **vitreous humour (Figure 1.12)**. This is a hydrated gel with fine collagenous fibres holding fluid to form a jelly-like structure. The jelly has several attachments to the retina. The strongest of these are around the optic nerve, on retinal blood vessels and at the anterior border of the retina in a region known as the **vitreous base.**

Uvea

The **uvea** is formed by the iris anteriorly and is continuous with the posterior aspect of the choroid, which underlies the retina. The choroid's function is to provide the highly metabolic retina with oxygenated blood and nutrition; consequently, the uvea is highly vascular and has one of the highest blood flows of any tissue.

Retina

The **retina** is a thin neurovascular layer composed of a multitude of specialised cells and is similar in thickness to tissue

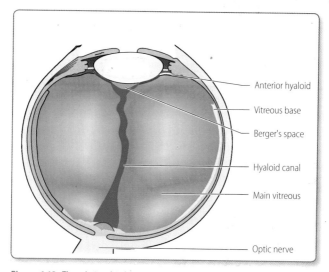

Figure 1.12 The relationship between the vitreous and ocular regions.

paper (**Figure 1.13a**). There are two types of **photoreceptors** (light-sensitive cells): **rods** and **cones** (**Figure 1.13b**). They are located in the outermost part of the neural retina. Rods are responsible for dim light vision and cones are responsible for colour vision in bright illumination.

Processing cells, found further in, include the horizontal and bipolar cells. These eventually synapse with ganglion cells. The unmyelinated axons of the retinal ganglion cells form the innermost layer of the retina – the nerve fibre layer. These axons course towards the **optic disc**, where they leave the eye through a perforation in the sclera to form the **optic nerve**.

The most sensitive portion of the retina with the greatest resolving capability is known as the **macula**. The most sensitive portion of the macula is the **fovea**, which is located between the upper and lower **temporal vascular arcades**.

1.2 Optics

The main refracting elements of the eye are:
- the cornea – fixed focus
- the crystalline lens – variable focus.

Accommodation is the process by which the eye is able to change its optical power in order to maintain focus at different distances. This is achieved through contraction of the **ciliary muscle**, which allows relaxation of the **zonular fibres** attached to the equatorial zone of the lens capsule (**Figure 1.14**).

Light transmission to the retina relies on transparent ocular media, which include the cornea, aqueous humour, lens and vitreous. These structures are devoid of blood vessels to maintain optical clarity. Since photoreceptors are found on the outer aspect of the neural retina, light must pass through the other retinal layers before being detected. Accommodation maintains clear focus of light rays in order to improve the definition of vision.

1.3 Physiology

Tear film

The tear film contains an inner proteinaceous layer, the main function of which is to adhere the tear film to the cornea.

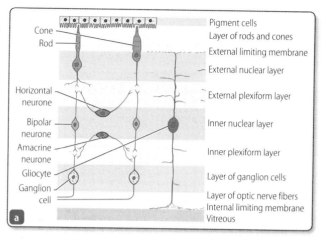

Pigment cells
Layer of rods and cones
External limiting membrane
External nuclear layer
External plexiform layer
Inner nuclear layer
Inner plexiform layer
Layer of ganglion cells
Layer of optic nerve fibers
Internal limiting membrane
Vitreous

Cone
Rod
Horizontal neurone
Bipolar neurone
Amacrine neurone
Gliocyte
Ganglion cell

a

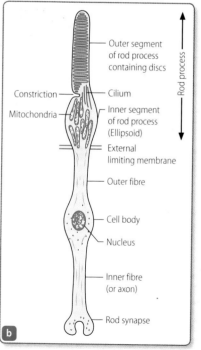

Outer segment of rod process containing discs
Cilium
Constriction
Mitochondria
Inner segment of rod process (Ellipsoid)
External limiting membrane
Outer fibre
Cell body
Nucleus
Inner fibre (or axon)
Rod synapse

Rod process

b

Figure 1.13 (a) Cellular structure of the retina. (b) Photoreceptor structure.

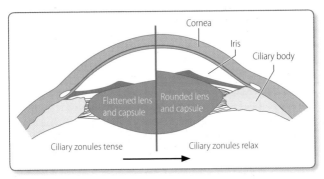

Figure 1.14 Changes in anatomy on accommodation.

The middle layer of the tear film is aqueous in nature, whereas the outer layer has a high lipid content in order to reduce tear evaporation (**Figure 1.15**). The spent tears are channelled towards two tiny orifices at the medial aspects of the eyelids, pass through their connecting tubes into the bridge of the nose and are flushed down the nasolacrimal duct into the nasopharynx.

Cornea

Increased hydration of the corneal stroma leads to disruption of the collagen fibril matrix causing loss of transparency of this tissue, which in health requires a tightly controlled hydration level. This dehydration is maintained by pumping fluid into the

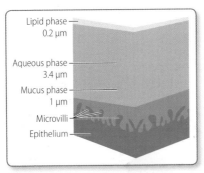

Figure 1.15 Pre-corneal tear film and lipid, aqueous and mucin components.

Lipid phase —
0.2 μm

Aqueous phase —
3.4 μm

Mucus phase —
1 μm

Microvilli —

Epithelium —

aqueous by corneal endothelial cells found on the innermost aspect of the cornea (**Figure 1.16**).

Aqueous

The aqueous humour, a watery but nutrient-rich liquid produced by the ciliary body, flows through the anterior part of the eye to the outflow at the angle between the cornea and the iris, known as the trabecular meshwork (**Figure 1.17**). The aqueous provides important nutrients to the avascular cornea and lens. Intraocular pressure is also manipulated by relative inflow or outflow of aqueous, a concept important to remember in understanding the pathogenesis and treatment of glaucoma.

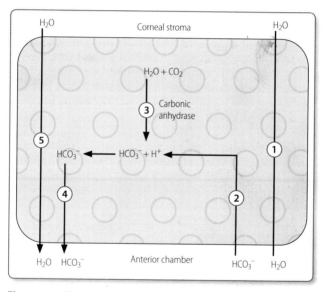

Figure 1.16 The endothelial pump generates a net ion movement from the stromal to anterior chamber side of the corneal endothelium. ① Passive diffusion into cell of H_2O. ② Passive diffusion into cell of HCO_3^-. ③ Carbonic anhydrase converts H_2O and CO_2 to HCO_3^- and H^+. ④ Anion-dependent ATPase. ⑤ H_2O passively follows bicarbonate to the aqueous-facing surface.

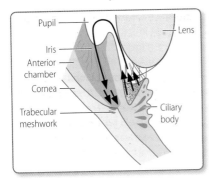

Figure 1.17 Aqueous flow from a ciliary process to the trabecular meshwork.

Lens

The outer capsule of the lens is attached to collagen fibrils known as **zonules** (**Figure 1.18**). These fibrils attach the lens to the ciliary body, which contains a circular and circumferentially arranged muscle. This apparatus permits some variability in focusing capability of the lens.

Clinical insight

The lens is an elastic structure. However, ageing leads to loss of elasticity, which can lead to problems with focusing, such as presbyopia.

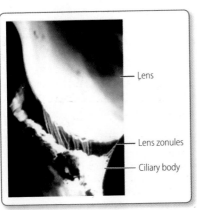

Figure 1.18 The lens and zonules.

Macula

Light falling upon the macula (**Figure 1.19**) serves a central visual function, such as reading. The highest resolving power is at the fovea. It is here that the finest blood vessels terminate in a **perifoveal vascular plexus** to support this highly metabolic neuroretinal tissue. The **foveal avascular zone** is the site at which light falls directly on the photoreceptor layer, with the overlying neuroretinal layers splayed to reveal a yellow dot visible with the ophthalmoscope. This **luteal pigment** is yellow to protect the central macula against photic damage.

Retinal pigment epithelium and Bruch's membrane (basal lamina of choroid)

Critical to the function of the photoreceptors is the **retinal pigment epithelium** (RPE) that separates the neuroretina from the underlying choroid (**Figure 1.20**). The basement of the RPE is known as the **Bruch's membrane** and is prone to

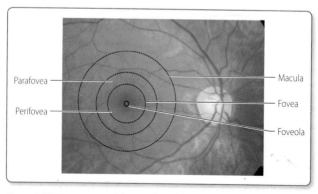

Figure 1.19 The structure of the macula and fovea.

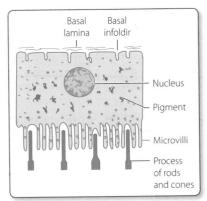

Figure 1.20 The photoreceptor and retinal pigment epithelial complex.

Labels in figure: Basal lamina, Basal infoldir, Nucleus, Pigment, Microvilli, Process of rods and cones

age-related changes affecting function. The RPE acts in a similar way to the blood–brain barrier and selectively allows chemicals in and out of the retina.

Below the RPE is the highly vascular choroid, which provides oxygen and nutrients to the highly metabolic retina as well as removing waste products. It is important that Bruch's membrane remains highly permeable for retinal homeostasis.

Clinical insight

Drusen are yellow/white deposits commonly seen in fundoscopy of people aged over 75. They are extracellular debris of photoreceptor metabolism deposited between the retinal pigment epithelium and Bruch's membrane. They accumulate with age and are thought to be involved in the pathogenesis of age-related macular degeneration. Drusen and other deposits reduce the permeability of Bruch's membrane and hence interfere with retinal homeostasis.

Ophthalmology in practice

All good clinicians are careful listeners, keen observers and demonstrate a logical approach to problem-solving. The information contained in this chapter will arm readers with the practical skills which will allow them to navigate their way along the diagnostic algorithms of the most commonly encountered clinical scenarios (see Chapter 3).

2.1 History taking

The common symptoms

The common symptoms encountered in the ophthalmic history are:

- visual disturbance
- double vision (diplopia)
- pain
- altered appearance
- wateriness (epiphora).

Each of the symptoms should be clarified as described below.

Visual disturbance

Monocular vs binocular

Monocular visual symptoms localise the lesion to the anterior visual pathways, i.e. the globe or optic nerve. **Binocular** symptoms result from posterior visual pathway lesions, i.e. optic chiasm, tracts, radiation or second eye involvement.

Positive vs negative scotoma

During the examination, the patient should be asked to describe the nature of the **scotoma** (blurred area). If the object is simply blurred, this is termed a positive scotoma and is more consistent with opacity in the ocular media (cornea, lens, vitreous) or a macular abnormality. If part of the blurred area is described as missing, this is termed a negative scotoma and is more consistent with an optic neuropathy or posterior visual pathway lesions.

Metamorphopsia

Metamorphopsia is the term used when objects appear distorted. If patients complain of blurring of central vision, they should be asked whether distortion is present. Distortion is highly suggestive of the presence of macular disease and is never present in optic nerve disease.

Flashing lights

Flashing lights denote the presence of irritation of the visual pathways, most commonly retinal traction, or, extremely rarely, a lesion in the occipital lobe.

Floaters

Floaters reflect opacities suspended in the vitreous gel, most commonly condensations of the vitreous but occasionally blood.

Glare

Glare is often associated with the presence of cataract.

Hallucinatory images

Hallucinatory images can often be associated with severe bilateral loss of vision, most commonly as a result of age-related macular degeneration. The patient is acutely aware that these images are spurious; this immediately differentiates them from hallucinations secondary to psychiatric disease. As patients are often reluctant to volunteer this information, they should be specifically asked whether they 'see images that are actually not there'.

Double vision (diplopia)
True diplopia vs blurred vision

If patients volunteer **diplopia** as a symptom, they should be immediately asked to clarify this as some patients use this term and blurred vision interchangeably.

Binocular vs monocular diplopia

If the patient confirms that he or she can see two separate objects (and not one blurred one), they should be asked to cover each eye in turn. If the diplopia disappears when each eye is covered in turn, the patient is describing binocular diplopia, which reflects a lack of coordination of eye movements. If the diplopia persists, the patient is describing monocular diplopia, which nearly always reflects the presence of cataract.

Pain
Sharp vs dull
The description of the character of the pain can help differentiate its cause:
- Pain arising from the surface of the eye, especially from the cornea, will usually be described as sharp
- Inflammation of the sclera or from within the eye will usually be described as dull
- Occasionally, the pain associated with acute angle closure glaucoma can be more marked above the eye

As a general rule, pain arising from the eye or the orbit will be associated with abnormalities found on clinical examination.

Photophobia

Photophobia is pain associated with light. It is a very useful diagnostic symptom associated with:
- inflammation arising in the eye (**iritis**)
- corneal inflammation (**keratitis**)
- rarely, ocular hypopigmentation (**albinism**)

Altered appearance

When this is volunteered by the patient or relative, it should be taken seriously as many patients are often unaware of even quite obvious changes in their appearance.

Wateriness (epiphora)

Epiphora is the term used for excessive wateriness in the eye. It can occur:

- in isolation, suggesting reduced drainage as the underlying cause
- with a foreign body sensation or itch, which is highly suggestive of ocular irritation and excessive tear production

<table>
<tr><td>

Guiding principle

- Each element of the history, examination and any investigation should answer, or at least help to answer, a diagnostic or therapeutic question
- The passive aspect of history taking can be improved by becoming a careful listener, and the active aspect can be improved by learning how to clarify the most frequently encountered ophthalmic symptoms

</td></tr>
</table>

Patients should be asked to clarify details of any past ocular problems/surgery. It is important to enquire about the patient's past medical and drug history and specifically tailor additional questions to the likely aetiology/risk factors relevant to the presenting complaint. It is important to determine whether there is any family history of eye disease.

2.2 Examination

The common signs

The common signs to look for in the ophthalmic examination are:

- blurred or distorted vision
- restricted visual fields
- facial asymmetry
- absence of normal structures, e.g. eyelashes
- presence of abnormal structures, e.g. tumours
- ocular inflammation
- haziness of ocular structures
- abnormal pupil reactions
- presence of a squint
- abnormal fundal appearance

Examination sequence

Senior clinicians will often perform only selected components of the clinical examination, using their experience to know what can be safely omitted. A suggested sequence for inexperienced clinicians is:

1. central vision (**visual acuity**)
2. peripheral vision (**visual fields**)
3. external eye
4. pupil reactions
5. cover test (if diplopia present)
6. fundoscopy

Visual acuity

Reduced visual acuity indicates opacity of the ocular media (cornea, lens, vitreous) or an abnormality of the visual pathways – most often the macula, less often the optic nerve. Visual acuity is always checked monocularly, with the patient having his or her refractive error corrected by glasses, contact lenses or a pinhole (see below).

Distance vision

Distance vision is measured using the **Snellen** (or equivalent) chart:

- The Snellen chart comprises letters of diminishing size that form a retinal image of similar size when viewed from a given distance from the chart, which is indicated by the number below any particular line
- The patient is positioned 6 m from the chart and instructed to read the smallest line he or she can see
- The result should be recorded, with the numerator being the test distance in metres (usually 6) and the denominator being the number below the smallest line of letters the patient is able to read
- If the patient cannot correctly identify 3 letters of the 6/18 line.

Eliminating refractive error

If the patient's visual acuity is reduced (i.e. less than 6/6), the test should be repeated with the patient looking through a **pinhole** to eliminate any refractive errors, such as myopia, hypermetropia or astigmatism, including the wearing of incorrect glasses. A few holes in a piece of card will suffice. If patients cannot read the largest letter (6/60), they should be asked, in the following order:

1. to count how many fingers you are holding up
2. whether they can perceive hand movements
3. whether they have any perception of light

If the patient is unable to see light, the patient is 'blind' and is classified as having no perception of light.

Near vision

The patient's **near vision** should be tested using the near-reading chart, which comprises a series of sentences of writing of standard size with the smallest type being denoted N5 and the largest N48. If the patient cannot read N5, the test should be repeated using the pinhole as above.

Supplementary tests of central vision

Supplementary tests of central vision include:

- testing colour vision using Ishihara plates
- testing redness/brightness perception
- an Amsler chart for detecting and documenting the presence of distortion

These can be useful both for differentiating optic nerve disease from macular disease and for detecting a change in ocular function over time.

Colour vision Ishihara produced a series of colour plates (**Figure 2.1**), each of which contains a circle of dots that appear

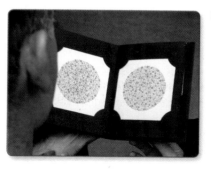

Figure 2.1 Ishihara plate.

to be randomised in colour and size. Within the pattern are dots that form a number visible to those with normal colour vision and invisible, or difficult to see, for those with either congenital (e.g. 1% of all males have an X-linked defect) or acquired red–green colour vision defects. A numerical score is given to the number of correct responses made by the patient. If a patient's colour vision is relatively more impaired than his or her visual acuity, it is more likely that the underlying cause will be an optic neuropathy rather than maculopathy.

Redness and brightness perception If Ishihara plates are unavailable, it is still useful to assess perception of redness and brightness. These tests are simple to perform and check the sensitivity of the central field to red targets and brightness of a light. The tests should be performed monocularly at the patient's normal reading distance:
- The patient is asked to look at a red target with each eye separately and to allocate a numerical score to the quality of the 'redness'
- The test is repeated but with a light source; the patient is asked to allocate a numerical score to the quality of the 'brightness'

Both these tests are most useful in the setting of unilateral symptoms/pathology when the 'redness' and 'brightness' can be directly compared between the affected and unaffected eyes:
- Starting with the unaffected eye, the patient is instructed to allocate a score of 5 for the eye's redness or brightness perception
- The abnormal eye is then examined by asking the patient to allocate the redness or brightness score themselves, with any reduction in either redness or brightness perception allocated a lower score
- A difference in the redness or brightness score between the two eyes indicates an underlying optic nerve disease or, as the optic nerve is made up of retinal cell axons, significant retinal disease

Amsler chart (Figure 2.2). This is a near-reading chart with a grid and a centrally placed fixation dot in place of letters;

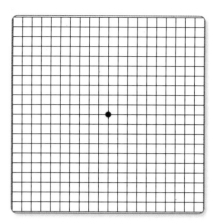

Figure 2.2 Amsler chart.

it is useful for eliciting the presence and extent of metamor-phopsia. The patient is asked to look at the fixation dot and to state whether or not any of the straight lines appear curved. It is useful to ask the patient to draw around the abnormal area; this can then be used to assess any change over time. The patient should also be asked whether any part of the chart is blurred or missing, as this will indicate the presence of a positive or negative scotoma.

> ## Guiding principle
>
> Supplementary tests of central vision, such as testing the redness/brightness perception and the use of the Amsler chart, can be useful in differentiating optic nerve disease from macular disease.

Visual fields

By 'mapping' the extent and shape of visual field defect in each eye separately, it should be possible to localise any lesion in the visual pathways. **Figure 2.3** demonstrates the typical visual field defects associated with lesions of the anterior and posterior visual pathways:

- The **anterior** pathways comprise the retina and optic nerve
- The **posterior** pathways comprise the optic chiasm, optic tracts and optic radiations (occipital lobe)

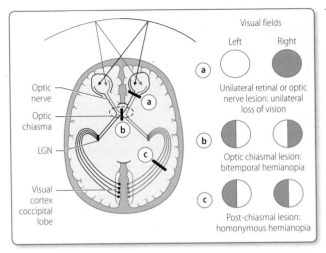

Figure 2.3 Visual pathway lesions and resultant visual field defects. Blue indicates the affected part of the visual field. LGN, lateral geniculate nucleus.

Disease of the retina or optic nerve head can be directly observed. In contrast, lesions that affect the posterior portion of the optic nerve or the posterior visual pathways cannot and their presence has to be inferred by the pattern of the patient's visual field loss.

Automated perimetry should be performed to document any visual field defects as this will allow subsequent comparisons to be made and changes reliably detected.

Confrontation visual field examination

Confrontation visual field testing provides vital and immediate diagnostic information. However, it will often only be possible to detect gross defects. As a clinician becomes more experienced in the technique, detection of more subtle defects becomes possible.

Visual fields should always be checked **monocularly**. The patient is instructed to cover one eye and look (fixate) at the bridge the examiner's nose at all times. If at any time the patient loses fixation, the test findings are inaccurate; if this happens, the test should be stopped and the patient should be reminded to maintain fixation.

The peripheral field of each eye is divided artificially into four quadrants – upper and lower, temporal and nasal – and each quadrant assessed separately:

1. Ask the patient 'can you see my face?' The patient may indicate that one half (upper or lower, right or left) of your face is missing
   - Monocular defects affecting either the upper or lower half of the visual field are often described as **altitudinal** and are particularly associated with vascular occlusions affecting the anterior visual pathways, either the retina or optic nerve head
   - Binocular defects of the right or left half of the visual field can be **homonymous** (same side) or **heteronymous** (opposite side; classically a bitemporal hemianopia, the hallmark of a chiasmal lesion) and point to a lesion of the patient's posterior visual pathways

2. Touch the patient's free hand and instruct him or her to point to which fingers they see moving. This bypasses the frequently encountered confusion of which side is being referred to

3. To test the peripheral visual field, place both of your hands into the centre of two diagonally opposite visual field quadrants (e.g. upper temporal and lower nasal) with your fingers at the peripheral limits of the patient's normal field (**Figure 2.4**)

4. Wiggle your fingers; if the patient sees the finger movement straight away, no further testing within the quadrant is necessary and it is deemed to be normal
   - If the patient is unable to detect the finger movement, continue finger wiggling while slowly moving the hand in a horizontal direction (**Figure 2.4**) towards the vertical

> ## Clinical insight
>
> To practise the correct initial hand positioning when testing visual fields, perform a confrontation visual field with a normally sighted colleague. Place your hands where you think they should be and hold still while the 'patient' moves your hands into the periphery of their normal visual field. In this way, practitioners become accustomed to the limits of a normal visual field.

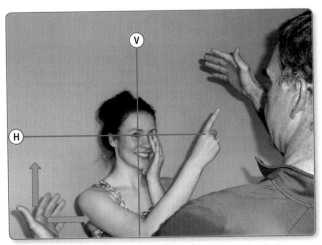

Figure 2.4 Confrontation visual field test demonstrating the correct initial positioning and subsequent movement of the examiner's hands (arrows). Ⓥ vertical meridian, Ⓗ horizontal meridian.

midline in order to ascertain the extent of the non-seeing area

- If the patient detects movement anywhere up to but not extending beyond the vertical midline then the visual field defect is said to respect the vertical meridian. This pattern, if bilateral, points to the lesion being located in the posterior visual pathways, i.e. it is **intracranial**

5. Next, place your hands back into the original starting position for that quadrant and move them in a vertical direction (**Figure 2.4**) to determine whether the visual field defect respects the horizontal midline

6. If the patient cannot detect finger movement but can perceive light, instruct the patient to 'look at my voice' while shining a light from each of the four quadrants in turn. Ask the patient to point to where the light is coming from. Quick and accurate projection of light indicates the integrity of the visual pathways. This test is often most useful in the setting of a patient with a very dense cataract and only perception of light

7. Examine the patient's other eye

Sensitivity of the central field to red targets

The sensitivity of the central field to red targets should be tested if a visual field defect cannot be demonstrated during confrontation testing but there is till suspicion of one being present:

> ### Guiding principle
>
> Patients presenting with loss of vision should have the extent and shape of their visual field defects delineated by confrontation testing to identify where in their visual pathways the lesion is located.

1. Instruct the patient to cover one eye and to fixate on the bridge of your nose.
2. Present a red target first just above then just below fixation, and ask the patient to comment on the relative redness of the target between above and below fixation as described above.
3. Repeat the same process, presenting the red object to the right and then to the left of fixation and ask the patient to make the same comparison

Interpretation: If the patient reports a difference in the perceived redness of the target either side of the horizontal meridian, suspect the presence of an anterior visual pathway lesion.

Conversely, if the patient perceives a difference either side of the vertical meridian bilaterally, suspect the presence of a posterior visual pathway lesion.

Mutlukan and Cullen red dots card

A particularly simple and clinically useful test of central colour vision is the Mutlukan and Cullen red dots card (**Figure 2.5**). This test is performed monocularly with the card at the patient's normal reading distance:

1. Ask the patient to fixate on the central black dot and comment on the presence and quality of the surrounding eight red dots
2. Pay particular attention to the quality of the patient's perception of the 'redness' of the dots either side of the vertical and horizontal meridians
3. If the patient reports the dots to be washed out, i.e. less vividly red in one hemi-field (vertical or horizontally separated) then

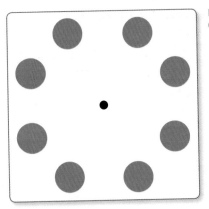

Figure 2.5 Mutlukan and Cullen red dots card.

interpret these results in exactly the same way as described above

External eye

The clinician will have made a general medical assessment of the patient's eyes whilst greeting them. After assessing the patient's vision, the temptation to examine the eye in isolation should be resisted; instead, it is better to pause and assess the patient's facial appearance.

Facial appearance

Abnormalities that are unilateral are always more easily observed than those that are bilateral and symmetrical; the detection of the latter relies more on the clinician's experience of what constitutes a deviation from the spectrum of normality.

Look for **asymmetry** between the two sides of the patient's face. If patients themselves have noted a change in their own appearance, due weight should be given to their own observations.

The eyes

A methodical assessment should be made of the position and size of the:
- globes
- eyelids

- pupils
- eyelashes
- sclerae and conjunctivae
- corneas

Globes The globes should be checked for proptosis, which is anterior displacement of the globe. This can be unilateral or bilateral, axial or non-axial. Axial proptosis is where the globe is displaced directly forwards, whereas in non-axial proptosis the globe is (also) displaced inferiorly, superiorly, medially or laterally. Common causes of globe displacement include:

- thyroid orbitopathy, the most commonly encountered cause of proptosis, which is **always** axial
- an enlarged lacrimal gland, causing inferomedial displacement
- fractures causing post-traumatic enophthalmos associated with subcutaneous emphysema and, occasionally, a 'step' felt on palpation of the orbital rim

Eyelids The normal resting position of the lower lid margin in most patients is touching the limbus (the junction between the peripheral cornea and the sclera) at the 6 o'clock position. The upper lid margin normally covers the superior 1–2 mm of the iris. Lids can be too low (ptosis) or too high (lid retraction or secondary to proptosis).

If the upper lid is abnormally high, inspection of the lower lid position helps to differentiate whether the cause is secondary to lid retraction or proptosis. Proptosis will be associated with lower lid retraction, which will be absent in cases of isolated upper lid retraction. Lids can also be:

- turned outwards (**ectropion**), which can be associated with **epiphora** (watering)
- turned inwards (**entropion**), when they will be associated with a foreign body sensation as the lashes scrape against the surface of the eye
- unable to close (**lagophthalmos**), seen by assessing the patient's blink and normal eyelid closure. Lagophthalmos will often be associated with more widespread facial asymmetry consistent with a facial nerve paralysis

Pupils A difference in pupil size is termed anisocoria. If ptosis is noted, it is important to check for the presence of anisocoria, which indicates an underlying neurogenic aetiology. On examination, a pupil can appear smaller, larger or irregular in shape:

- A small pupil (**miosis**) in conjunction with ipsilateral ptosis of 1–2 mm can be associated with **Horner syndrome** (oculosympathetic palsy) resulting from a cervical or thoracic sympathetic chain lesion
- A dilated pupil (**mydriasis**), when associated with ptosis of any severity or disorder of eye movements, indicates the presence of an **oculomotor** (third nerve) palsy
- An irregular-shaped pupil can reflect trauma (sphincter tears) or adhesions (synechiae) at the pupil margin, or rarely dialysis of the root of the iris from the sclera. A peaked pupil following a sharp injury is highly suggestive of a penetrating injury

Eyelashes Checks should be made for structures which are normally present, e.g. eyelashes – their focal absence will often be associated with eyelid margin neoplasia (most commonly a basal cell carcinoma). It is also important to look for lesions which should not be present, such as xanthelasma (fatty deposits on the eyelids) and abnormal pigmentation.

Sclerae and conjunctivae These structures should be examined principally for the presence of inflammation, in particular if it is present bilaterally or unilaterally. If unilateral, a note should be made of whether the inflammation is present diffusely or only in one sector. If sectorial, the redness should be regarded as an arrow pointing at the adjacent peripheral cornea. If the cornea is normal, the sectorial redness is likely to be due to scleritis or episcleritis. The distinction between limbal (the junction of the sclera and cornea) and peripheral redness is of arguable diagnostic value.

Cornea If the cornea is described as clear or hazy in appearance:
- focal haze is the hallmark of stromal (middle layer of the cornea) **keratitis** (inflammation of the cornea)

- generalised haze sometimes reflects diffuse corneal oedema, only seen as a late manifestation of acute angle closure glaucoma

Fluorescein sodium dye is used to confirm the presence of epithelial keratitis, as it fills the corneal defect, absorbs blue light and glows green. This is particularly important in the presence of an inflamed eye or a 'white eye' that is painful. Subtle abnormalities of the cornea can be made more obvious with magnification. If a slit lamp is not available, the direct ophthalmoscope can be used as a strong illuminated magnifier.

Slit lamp examination

The ocular examination, as described above, assumes that a slit lamp is not available. The observations are just as valid if one is available and you are competent to use it. The slit lamp confers many advantages over simple observation with a light source, the two most important being the high degree of magnification and illumination. The anterior chamber, lens and anterior vitreous can be directly viewed and, with the aid of special lenses, the retinal structures can observed.

Pupil reactions

The key clinical examination is the swinging flashlight test, which will elicit the presence of a **relative afferent pupil defect** (RAPD). A RAPD is associated with optic nerve disease or, as the optic nerve comprises retinal ganglion cell axons, with retinal pathology affecting more than a third of the retina.

Swinging flashlight test

This test should be conducted in dim lighting conditions with a strong light source and the patient looking at a distant target. These factors ensure the greatest amplitude of pupil excursion, facilitating the detection of a RAPD. The most important element of the technique is, after noting the initial reaction of the pupil, to swing the light as fast as possible between the patient's eyes:

1. Ask the patient to focus on a distal point; note the size of the pupils in the dim lighting conditions

2. From about 10 cm away from the eye being tested, first shine the pen torch into one eye and note the initial reaction of the pupil to the light

3. After noting the initial reaction of the pupil, swing the light as fast as possible between the two eyes and note the initial reaction of the other pupil

4. A RAPD is present if, when the swinging light shines into the patient's eye, the pupil paradoxically dilates. The absence of a constriction also indicates the presence of a RAPD

This test can still be conducted in the presence of only one mobile pupil:

- Perform the technique as above but observe the reaction of only the mobile pupil
- If the mobile pupil dilates when the light is shining into the contralateral eye, the presence of a RAPD is confirmed in that eye

A slit lamp can be used to observe a sighted eye with a pupil that fails to contract to light. The iris may be atrophic (iris transillumination will be observed), hence too weak to react, or, rarely, it may be mechanically prevented from contracting by the presence of significant **synechiae** (adhesions between the iris and lens secondary to inflammation). If neither abnormality is noted, the slit should be reduced to the height of the pupil and shone directly through it.

The hallmark of an **Adie pupil** (post-ganglionic parasympathetic paresis) is the uncoordinated 'vermiform' (snake like) segmental contractions of sections of the iris, which, if present, are pathognomonic.

Lastly, the effect of reading a paragraph (a practical way of testing the near response) on the unreactive pupil should be noted.

Light–near dissociation occurs when a pupil fails to constrict to light but does so for near focusing (i.e. accommodation); this demonstrates light–near dissociation and indicates a midbrain lesion.

> **Guiding principle**
>
> The key test of optic nerve function is the swinging flashlight test to elicit the presence of a relative afferent pupil defect.

Cover test

A cover test confirms the presence of an ocular deviation and is most useful in the context of diplopia with no squint obvious. It cannot be carried out in a blind eye or without the cooperation of the patient.

The patient should be instructed to look at a fixation target the examiner is holding, and asked to cover each eye in turn:

- If, when one eye is covered, the other eye moves to take up fixation, the uncovered eye must have been squinting
- If it moves outwards, it must have been inturning; if it moves downwards, it must have been upturning; and so on
- If the uncovered eye fails to move, no squint is present

The alternate cover test is used to check the maximum deviation. This is performed by alternately blocking fixation between the patient's eyes.

Fundoscopy

Fundoscopy is the examination of the retina using an ophthalmoscope. Unless the pupil is dilated with a short-acting mydriatic agent (dilating drop) such as tropicamide 1.0% or 0.5%, it is unlikely that anything will be seen in the fundus (retina) other than the optic disc. The tiny risk of inducing angle closure glaucoma has to be balanced against the much more likely risk of failing to view the fundus well enough if dilating drops are not used.

Procedure

1. Ask the patient to remove his or her glasses. Occasionally, if the patient wears very thick glasses you may see the fundus better if the glasses remain worn, but always try without first
2. Set the ophthalmoscope focusing dial to zero, or the appropriate setting to correct your refractive error
3. Ask the patient to focus on a distant target
4. Stand 1 m from the patient to check for the presence and quality of the red reflex. This is the light reflected back through the pupil

Guiding principle

Fundoscopy should be performed using a light beam of the least intensity and the smallest diameter that allows visualisation of the fundus.

- A reduced red reflex is associated with opacities in the ocular structures (media) that the light rays pass through. From front to back, this includes the cornea, lens, vitreous and retina

5. To visualise the patient's right fundus, use your right eye and hold the ophthalmoscope in your right hand; to visualise the patient's left eye, use your left eye and hold the ophthalmoscope in your left hand

6. Move the ophthalmoscope in, directing the light through the pupil at about 45° nasally, which usually results in the optic disc being visualised. If not, bring a blood vessel into focus by turning the lens dial and follow it until the disc is visible. Describe the optic disc in terms of:
   - **m** – sharpness of the disc margin
   - **c** – colour of the neuroretinal rim
   - **c** – cup, which is the ratio of the vertical height of the central cup to the overall vertical disc diameter

The retina

The retina is divided into a central macula (bounded by the temporal arcades) and the peripheral retina. It is important to look for:
- the foveal reflex in younger patients
- haemorrhages
- exudates
- abnormal pigmentation

The macula should be viewed first, with particular attention being paid to the appearance of the fovea. If the fovea cannot be identified, instruct the patient to cover his or her other eye and look into the light; this will identify the fovea. Lastly, the peripheral retina should be examined.

An ophthalmoscope may have the facility to change the colour of the light beam to either blue or green. Fluorescein dye will absorb light of blue wavelength and reflect back light of green wavelength, which facilitates the detection of corneal epithelial defects. Green (red free) light highlights blood as black, making haemorrhages and blood vessels more recognisable.

2.3 Investigations

One of the many attractions of ophthalmology is the clinician's ability to directly observe the signs of disease. There are, therefore, very few specialist investigations that are of particular relevance to the junior clinician. However, simple investigations are sometimes required to identify risk factors for patients with an established diagnosis (e.g. blood pressure and urinalysis in patients with vascular occlusions).

Ophthalmological investigations generally measure the structure and function of the patient's eye(s); these are then compared with the contralateral eye in unilateral disease and with an age-matched normal range. Changes in structure can be detected when the patient's appearance is compared over a series of visits. This is commonly accomplished by the use of clinical photography or by more specialised imaging techniques, including optical coherence tomography (OCT), ultrasound and fundus fluorescein angiogram (FFA). The most commonly used test of function is automated visual field testing (perimetry).

Imaging
Optical coherence tomography

OCT is a non-invasive investigation that uses the reflectance of infrared rays to provide structural information about the eye. Although initially intended for retinal investigation, OCT is increasingly being used for other ocular structures, including investigation of the retinal nerve fibre layer, cornea, iris and angle in glaucoma.

Ultrasound

Ultrasound uses an electric current to produce a vibration in a piezoelectric crystal in order to generate ultrasound waves. Machines measure the reflectance of sound waves at the interfaces of different structures to develop an interpretable picture of the eye.

An A-scan ultrasound measures the reflectance in just one plane, whereas a B-scan measures the reflectance in various planes to produce a two-dimensional image of the eye. An A-scan is most commonly used to measure the length of the eye prior to cataract surgery to calculate intraocular lens power. A B-scan is primarily used to provide structural information about the eye when the view is obscured.

Fundus fluorescein angiogram

A FFA is an invasive investigation of the vascular supply of the retina and choroid. Fluorescein is injected intravenously and arrives within the eye within seconds. When fluorescein is exposed to a light of approximately 494 nm wavelength, it fluoresces in yellow (521 nm). A FFA allows serial visualisation of the retinal circulation with the use of a camera with appropriate filters.

A FFA is most commonly used to look for retinal vascular abnormalities such as poor perfusion in ischaemic diabetic disease or new vessels from the choroid in age-related macular degeneration.

2.4 Diagnosis

Referral

For non-ophthalmic doctors and optometrists, the most important aspect of management is to establish a clinical diagnosis and to decide whether the patient requires referral to the ophthalmologist and, if so, how quickly.

Caution in diagnosis

One of the pitfalls is to succumb to the temptation to make a diagnosis without all of the information required to do so. From both the patient's and the clinician's perspective it is much safer to list a differential diagnosis and to state that any particular symptom, sign or investigation remains 'unexplained'. This ensures that your mind and, more importantly, that of the next person to assess the patient remains open to the underlying cause of the symptoms. If the patient's condition does not respond in the way expected with or without intervention, it is important to question the diagnosis.

Associated and underlying disease

Once the diagnosis is established, the presence of any local or systemic associations should be determined, e.g. an increased incidence of optic gliomas and phaeochromocytomas in patients with type 1 neurofibromatosis. It is important to be pragmatic, excluding treatable causes for disease, e.g. compression/avitaminosis in optic neuropathies. If the disease is untreatable, identification and amelioration of associated risk factors should be attempted to help reduce the risk of second eye involvement. An example of this is that an arteritic aetiology underlying an anterior ischaemic optic neuropathy carries a 50% risk of contralateral eye involvement in the absence of appropriate treatment.

2.5 Treatment

Broadly speaking, management can be divided into observation and intervention:

- **Observation** is an active process and involves the detection of change in appearance and/or function over time. The ocular structures can be affected by a wide variety of pathological processes, including infection, inflammation and vascular occlusion
- **Interventions** can be medical or surgical, and both benefit from the ease by which the eye is accessed. Abnormalities of both the ocular surface and the superficial structures can usually be treated using topical agents to ensure that a larger proportion of the treatment reaches the target structures and less enters the circulation

Intervention options include:

- *Topical treatment*: drops can be used to treat abnormalities of the conjunctiva, cornea, iris and ciliary body, but they do not penetrate more deeply
- *Systemic treatment*: abnormalities of the vitreous, choroid and retina require systemically administered treatment or, alternatively, are treated by drug injections into the vitreous cavity
- *Surgical interventions*, often using lasers, are indicated in the restoration of the clarity, shape or position of the ocular structures

Ocular pharmacology

Although the eye may be accessible to detailed examination, its internal structures, including the retina and optic nerve, are well protected by design. Topically applied drops (**Figure 2.6**) or ointments, which are the most common ways of delivering drugs to the eye, must overcome the eye's natural defences. Other modes of delivery are oral or intravenous preparations for systemic medications, and intravitreal and periocular injection for localised delivery.

Barriers to drug delivery

The main barriers to drug delivery are:
- compliance
- poor technique
- short residence time
- wash-out from tears

External eye barriers to drug delivery The eye's barriers include lids, tear outflow and ocular wall structure and are major obstacles to

> **Clinical insight**
>
> Sending copies of clinical letters to the patient helps them understand their own eye condition and its treatment. It also allows direct phone contact between the patient and the practitioner to clarify diagnosis, treatment and referral.
>
> Eye care is increasingly being shared between the hospital eye service and the patient's optician. Specific instructions can be given regarding re-referral and for both these reasons a copy letter should also always be sent to the patient's optician.

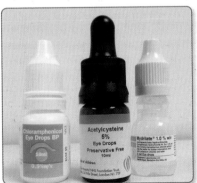

Figure 2.6 An eyedrop bottle.

externally applied drugs being delivered to the target tissue for prolonged periods. One of the first barriers is the tear film, which diluted topically applied medications with each blink (**Figure 2.7**).

Compliance Patient compliance with eyedrop treatments influences therapeutic outcome; it is important to spend time explaining the rationale, technique and expected result to patients and their accompanying family or friend.

Physical barriers to compliance include:
· poor vision
· arthritic fingers
· severe kyphosis leading to inability to self-instil medication
Cognitive decline and poor memory will also limit the patient's compliance. When treatment with drops is for a limited period and produces symptomatic improvement, e.g. in acute iritis, motivation to comply with therapy is usually good. For conditions that are chronic, painless and in which treatment is aimed at preventing rather than curing disease, such as open angle glaucoma, compliance is less good. A range of aides-memoire, gadgets (such as autodroppers) to ease instillation and regular consultation may be needed.

Drug design

Drug formulation The formulation or composition of the drug is determined by its physicochemical characteristics. For example, pH and solubility of the chemical predicts the nature

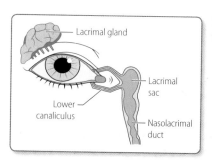

Figure 2.7 Tear (lacrimal) production and outflow.

Lacrimal gland

Lacrimal sac

Lower canaliculus

Nasolacrimal duct

of the vehicle in which it is prepared. The molecular size and solubility will affect drug passage and residence time within and across the corneal epithelium, stroma and endothelium; this is an important consideration for those drugs that need to access the anterior chamber to achieve their desired effect.

Crossing the cornea In treating both iritis and glaucoma, for example, the medication must cross the cornea in order to reach the aqueous humour and ciliary body, respectively. To do this, it must have both water- and lipid-soluble characteristics. Lipid solubility is required in order to pass the epithelium and endothelium, and water solubility is required to pass the stroma.

Efficacy The affinity, specificity and binding capabilities of the individual drugs used will determine their effectiveness. The clearance mechanisms both outside and inside the eye will shape the systemic side-effect profile and duration of action.

Drops and ointments

For patients with an extremely dry eye surface, artificial tear drops may be needed very frequently when evaporation loss adds to the fleetingly short effect of each instillation. Thicker, more viscous, preparations may be retained longer, but may cause blurring. Blocking the puncti, the orifices of tear outflow in the eyelids, with miniature plugs (**Figure 2.8**) may assist drop preservation on the eye surface.

Eyedrop toxicity Worsening ocular symptoms despite eyedrop treatment should raise suspicions of toxicity arising from the therapy (**Figure 2.9**). This is often associated with the preservatives and vehicles used in eyedrop preparations.

> ## Clinical insight
>
> When prescribing drops, it is important to tell patients to keep their eyes shut for 30 s following instillation of the drops to ensure effective absorption. Ointments used at night last longer than drops and will not be associated with blurring of the vision.

Periocular injection

Periocular injection is used when deeper penetration and a more sustained impact is required, e.g. in chronic ocular

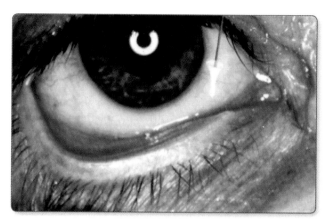

Figure 2.8 Punctal plug insertion.

inflammation. A bolus of drug is delivered beneath the conjunctiva but external to the sclera. The route of entry of drugs is both transcleral and intravenous from systemic absorption of the injected bolus by periocular vessels.

Intravitreal injection

Intravitreal injection utilises a sharp needle to pierce the sclera and deliver drugs to the vitreous from externally. This is now the mainstay of drug delivery for:

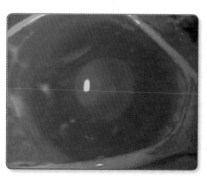

Figure 2.9 Punctate keratopathy with fluorescein.

- antineovascular drugs in macular degeneration
- long-term intraocular corticosteroids
- antibiotic treatment of intraocular infection

Although better for control of concentrations of drugs with intraocular effect, benefits have to be balanced alongside complications with this approach; these include:

- intraocular infection
- retinal toxicity
- retinal detachment

Oral and intravenous dosing

Oral dosing is the preferred option for patients with bilateral disease or systemic disease. For example, oxytetracycline tablet formulation is used in the treatment of chronic blepharitis associated with rosacea.

Corticosteroids are often prescribed orally in bilateral or chronic **uveitis**, an inflammation of the uveal tract. Occasionally, even parenteral drug delivery may be required to treat sight-threatening orbital inflammatory disease, optic neuritis and retinal infection. Effective prescribing requires an understanding of the systemic side-effects as well as the ocular benefits.

Side-effects

All drugs have side-effects. Balancing risk versus benefit is important in prescribing practice. For example, beta-blocker eye drops are a common treatment for glaucoma, yet they can cause systemic difficulties, including asthma and impotence. Side-effects can affect compliance; it is always helpful to discuss potential common and serious side-effects with patients before prescribing drugs.

Diagnostic algorithms

Experienced examiners use a number of decision-making strategies for diagnosis and treatment, including simple pattern recognition and the use of probabilities. Deductive medical reasoning is the process by which the diagnosis is established by analysing the presenting symptom or sign using a sequence of questions or observations that usually have a binomial response, such as 'yes/no' or 'present/absent'.

This chapter outlines a series of questions or observations pertaining to the most commonly encountered clinical scenarios. These algorithms, or decision trees, are the written framework of the deductive procedure that experienced examiners use to streamline the diagnostic process. Inexperienced observers will quickly become confident and competent in the clinical application of these basic algorithms and will be in a position to add new elements that will allow them to differentiate a greater number of diagnostic possibilities. Note that the focus of this chapter is on diagnostic, and not therapeutic, algorithms.

The diagnostic algorithms in this chapter cover the following topics:
- red eye(s) (**Figure 3.1**)
- loss of vision (**Figure 3.2**)
- double vision (diplopia) (**Figure 3.3**)
- watery eye(s) (epiphora) (**Figure 3.4**)
- pupils of different sizes (anisocoria) (**Figure 3.5**)

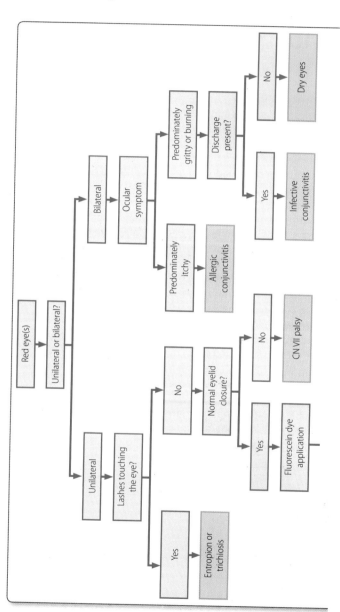

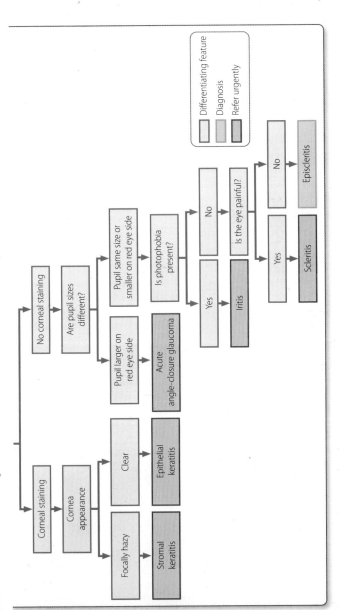

Figure 3.1 Red eye – diagnostic algorithm.

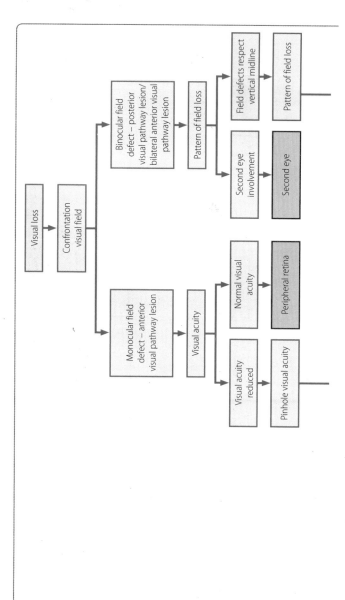

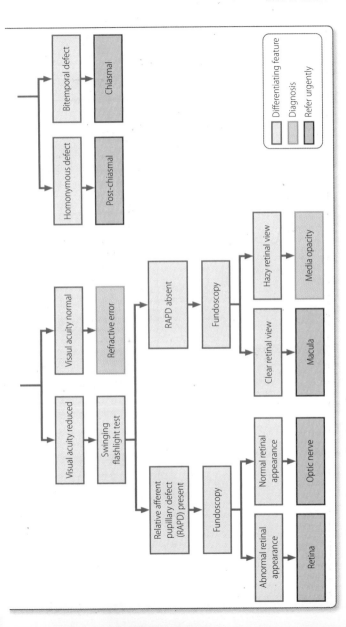

Figure 3.2 Loss of vision – diagnostic algorithm.

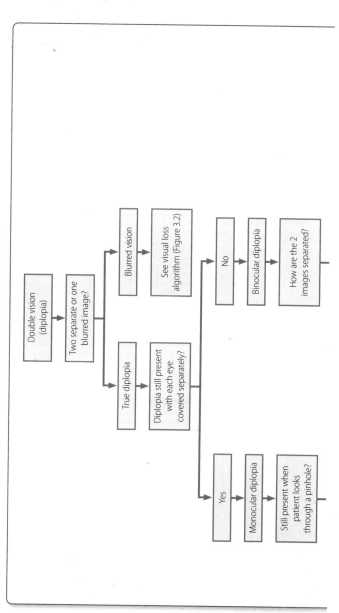

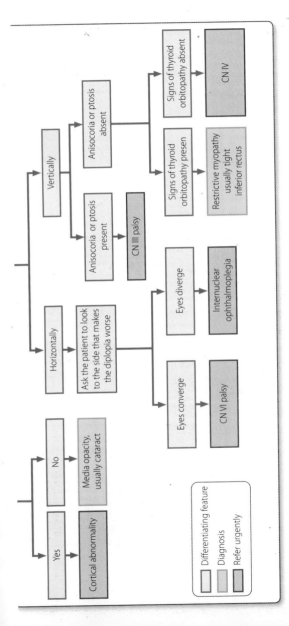

Figure 3.3 Double vision – (diplopia) diagnostic algorithm.

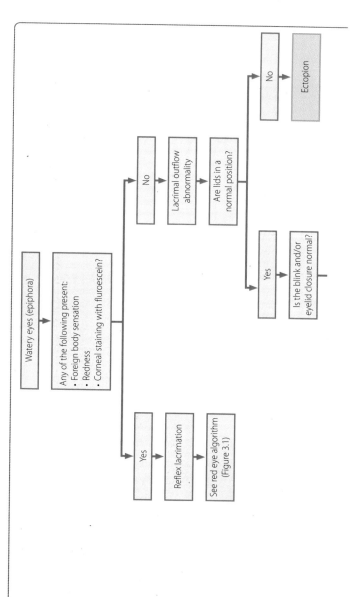

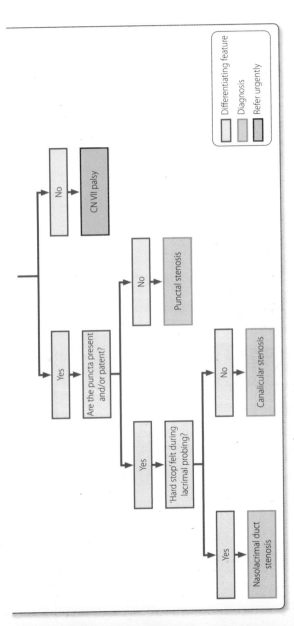

Figure 3.4 Watery eye(s) (epiphora) – diagnostic algorithm.

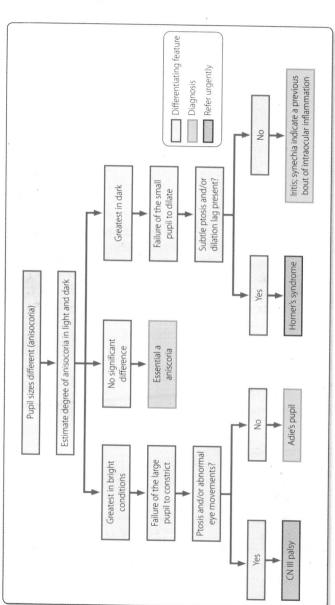

Figure 3.5 Pupils of different sizes (anisocoria) – diagnostic algorithm.

Refractive apparatus

Refractive errors are the commonest cause of blindness in the world. The number of people with refractive errors is also increasing worldwide. The majority of disorders can be easily treated by spectacle correction. Increasingly, contact lens wear, laser refractive surgery and intraocular lens replacement is being used for correction of all types of refractive error.

Anatomy and physiology

Refraction is a manifestation of the refracting components of the eye (the cornea, aqueous humour, lens and vitreous humour), their refractive indices (affected, for example, by curvature) and the length of the eye. Refractive errors occur when the eye is unable to focus incoming light rays onto the retina and can be due to any of these elements. Most commonly, it results from differences in corneal shape and eye axial length.

4.1 Clinical scenario

Gradually blurring vision

Presentation

A 55-year-old man presents to the outpatient department of his local hospital complaining of gradually increasing blurred vision.

Diagnostic approach

It is important to clarify initially whether the patient has true blurring with reduced visual acuity reduction or whether he has double vision.

Diagnostic clues in the history The patient states that the loss of vision is gradual and bilateral. Bilateral blurred vision will either have a systemic disease/change that affects both eyes or a single defect affecting the visual pathway beyond the chiasm. It is only very rarely that a disease affecting one eye will also simultaneously affect the other eye, e.g. retinal detachment or retinal vein occlusion.

Gradual onset helps rule out certain conditions such as vascular disorders. The next characteristic to make clear is whether the loss of vision affects the whole of his visual field or only part of it. The latter is more likely to point towards a defect in the visual pathway beyond the chiasm (see **Table 4.1** for causes).

Further history

The patient states that his vision is actually reduced with no double vision. This seems to occur only when reading and has recently also been worsening when working at his computer and affects all of his vision. Distance vision is unaffected. He has no other symptoms.

Previous medical history The patient reports that he has been diagnosed with hypertension.

Previous ocular history There is no previous ocular history of note. The patient does not wear glasses and he has not attended an opticians for some time.

Medications The patient takes bendroflumethiazide for hypertension.

Cause	Disease
Refractive	Myopia: difficulty with distance vision Hypermetropia: difficulty with near vision Astigmatism: distance and near blurry
Corneal	Corneal degeneration: corneal opacity and occasionally recurrent erosions and foreign body sensation
Lens	Cataract: glare Presbyopia: difficulty with near vision but not distance if refraction is correct
Retinal	Retinal degeneration, e.g. retinitis pigmentosa Dark adaptation, partial loss of field
Postchiasmal	Tumour: other neurological signs, partial field loss

Table 4.1 Differential diagnoses for gradual bilateral loss of vision.

Social history The patient is an accountant and a non-smoker.

Diagnostic approach

The fact that the vision loss covers most of the field of vision removes the risk of **postchiasmal disorders** (i.e. defects caused by interruption of pathways after the chiasm). The clue in the history is the intermittent nature of visual blurring. The patient states that the deficit only occurs when viewing near items. This means that a global reduction in vision, e.g. due to cataract, is eliminated, leaving only an accommodation defect such as **presbyopia**, a defect in accommodation with age, as a possible cause.

Examination

The results of a general examination were normal.

Ophthalmic examination For further information on the ophthalmic clinical examination, see **Table 4.2**.

Diagnostic approach

The examination seems normal except for the disparity between near and distance. The patient states that he has not been

Right eye		Left eye
6/6 N24	**Visual acuity** **Unaided distance** **Near**	6/6 N24
No response to direct and consensual light	**Pupil**	Normal response to direct and consensual light
Clear	**Cornea**	Clear
Clear	**Anterior chamber**	Clear
Clear	**Lens**	Clear
Clear	**Vitreous**	Clear
Clear view of fundus	**Fundus**	Clear view of fundus
Normal	**Disc**	Normal

Table 4.2 Ophthalmic examination: results for a patient who presented with gradually blurring vision

to the opticians in some time, which means that his refractive correction has not been checked recently. When accommodation reduces with age, this suggests presbyopia.

4.2 Hypermetropia

Hypermetropia, or far sightedness, is a refractive error in which parallel light rays entering the eye are focused beyond the retina (**Figure 4.1**). It is denoted by the (+) symbol, meaning that positive diopteric powered lenses (converging lenses) are required to correct the error.

Epidemiology

Hypermetropia is more common in children, partly because they have a shorter eye. At birth, on average a child is +2 dioptres in power. This reduces with time and, as a child's eyes grows longer, they become more emmetropic. Afro-Caribbean populations have an increased prevalence of hypermetropia, whereas East Asian populations have a reduced prevalence.

Clinical features

The clinical features of hypermetropia include:
- blurry vision
- headache, as the eye constantly accommodates to try to maintain retinal focus

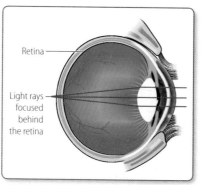

Figure 4.1 The convergence of incoming light behind the retina in a patient with hypermetropia.

Retina

Light rays focused behind the retina

Clinically, hypermetropia can be divided into physiological, pathological and functional causes (**Table 4.3**).

Diagnostic criteria

Please see **Table 4.4** for the classification of hypermetropia.

Risks

The risks of hypermetropia include **acute angle closure glaucoma** as hypermetropes generally have shorter eyes and therefore a more occludable drainage angle (see Chapter 12).

Hypermetropia also increases the risk of a convergent squint and, in children, there is a risk of **amblyopia**, which is developmental suppression of vision (see Chapter 14).

Type of hypermetropia	Causes	Clinical features
Physiological	Variation of normal Hereditary Flatter cornea Thinner lens Shorter eye	Blurry vision Headache or pain using eyes Squint Amblyopia
Pathological	Developmental eye abnormality to cornea and lens Acquired damage, e.g. trauma	Generalised systemic abnormalities History of trauma
Functional	Presbyopia (section 4.5) resulting in lack of accommodation	Older than 40 years Blurry vision and headaches with near work

Table 4.3 Clinical classification of hypermetropia

Description	Power (dioptres)
Low	< +2.25
Moderate	+2.25 to +5.00
High	> +5.00

Table 4.4 Classification of severity of hypermetropia

Investigations

In children, retinoscopy with a cycloplegic agent, which blocks accommodation, allows measurement of the refractive power. Normal retinoscopy and subjective correction can be performed in adults. Investigations should also include a review of ocular motility to rule out any squint and a full eye examination.

Differential diagnosis

The differential diagnoses include:
- other causes of reduced vision (see **Figure 3.2**)
- in adults, rarely, a raised retina, e.g. because of a tumour

Management

The decision whether to treat hypermetropia and how it is to be treated depends on a number of factors. These include the patient's age, symptomatology, power of the other eye, whether amblyopia is present and whether there is an associated squint. Low hypermetropia does not need to be treated if the patient has no symptoms and there is no other abnormality with both eyes. Otherwise, treatment should be given initially with full refractive correction. This can take many forms, including glasses, contact lenses and increasingly, in adults, laser surgery.

Prognosis

In the majority of children, their eyes become less hypermetropic with age, normalising by the age of 5–10 years. Children with amblyopia or squint are less likely to achieve full binocular vision.

Adult physiological hypermetropia is easily treated with refractive correction. Pathological refraction has a worse final visual prognosis owing to anatomical disruption to ocular structures.

4.3 Myopia

Myopia, or short sightedness, results when parallel rays of light entering the eye have a focal point short of the retina (**Figure 4.2**). This is caused by a combination of the refractive

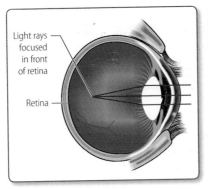

Light rays
focused
in front
of retina

Retina

Figure 4.2 Convergence of incoming light to a focal point in front of the retina in a patient with myopia.

components of the eye and the length of the eye. It is denoted by the (–) symbol, meaning that a divergent or negative lens is required to correct the condition.

Epidemiology

Myopia is one of the most common causes of treatable blindness in the world. The prevalence of myopia varies from region to region. In South East Asian countries, the prevalence may be as high as 80%; in Western Europe, it is 40%; and in some African countries, it is as low as 10%. Myopia is rare in children, although it is more commonly found in those born prematurely. Prevalence increases with age as the infant's eye grows longer.

Causes

Myopia has a large hereditary component. Several genes have now been identified that cause high myopia. How much early visual experience plays in this has yet to be determined, but there is a link between myopia, academia and occupation.

Pathogenesis

During early childhood, the eye gradually becomes more myopic in a process known as emmetropisation. This results from a balance between the eye growing longer and the cornea flattening. In some cases, this process continues beyond **emmetropia** –

normal vision – leading to the development of myopia. In a small minority, the development of myopia progresses throughout life. The exact mechanism is unknown, but genes are thought to play a large part in setting the range of myopia, with childhood visual activity adjusting the level of final myopia.

Other causes of myopia include pathology such as changes to the refractive components of the eye, which can be congenital or acquired. Congenital causes include genetic or developmental conditions such as Down syndrome. Acquired causes include cataract, which results from increased lens refractive power and, therefore, shortening of the focal length. In addition, trauma to the cornea or lens can result in myopia by alteration to the optical components of the eye.

Clinical features

The main clinical feature of myopia is blurry vision, especially for distance.

Diagnostic criteria

Please see **Table 4.5** for the classification of severity of myopia.

Risks

Patients with myopia have an increased risk of retinal detachment and macular degeneration. The reduced trabecular meshwork aqueous flow and weakness of the optic nerve head in myopia increase the risk of **open angle glaucoma** (see Chapter 12).

> **Clinical insight**
>
> A pinhole can correct visual acuity by up to three lines on the Snellen chart and is useful to estimate full corrected vision if a patient's glasses are not available.

Description	Dioptres of myopia
Low myopia	< −3.25
Moderate myopia	−3.25 to −6.00
High myopia	> −6.00

Table 4.5 Classification of severity of myopia

Investigations

As with all causes of reduced vision, it is important to obtain a full history and examination. It is also important to assess visual acuity to rule out any sinister causes of myopia, such as trauma. You should give special consideration to asymmetric myopia.

Management

Patient factors are important in deciding whether to treat myopia. Treatment is not necessary if patients are asymptomatic, e.g. in low myopia, except in amblyopia (see Chapter 14); however, the decision should take account of considerations such as driving and occupation (aviation, military, police and driving heavy goods vehicles).

Spectacle correction is still the most important form of correction, with contact lens and corneal laser surgery gaining popularity.

> **Clinical insight**
>
> Refractive correction does not reduce the risk of associated problems (glaucoma, retinal detachment, degeneration).

Prognosis

The prognosis is generally good for moderate and low myopia. However, with every dioptre greater than −8, the risk of retinal detachment (see Chapter 11) and myopic degeneration increases markedly.

4.4 Astigmatism

The focus of incoming light rays into the eye is mainly affected by the cornea and the lens. Most commonly, the cornea is round like a football. However, in astigmatism, the cornea is more like a rugby ball, and light rays entering the eye at different points of the cornea are focused differently depending on where they enter the cornea (**Figure 4.3**). This results in a blurred retinal image. A cylindrical lens is required to correct this abnormality.

Epidemiology

Approximately one third of people have some kind of astigmatism.

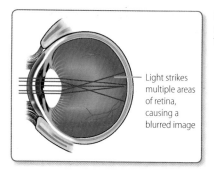

Figure 4.3 Focusing parallel light rays entering the eye in astigmatism.

Light strikes multiple areas of retina, causing a blurred image

Causes

Astigmatism is most commonly a result of irregular corneal curvature. A rare form of abnormal corneal curvature is a condition called keratoconus, an ectasia of the cornea that results in marked astigmatism. The lens occasionally causes astigmatism as a result of irregularities in its surface. Trauma or surgery can both result in astigmatism by causing irregular shaping of the cornea or misaligning the lens.

Pathogenesis

Astigmatism is mainly hereditary. The exceptions are the acquired causes affecting corneal curvature.

Clinical features

The clinical features of astigmatism include:
· blurred vision
· headaches

Investigations

A full ophthalmic examination should be carried out. The patient's visual acuity should be assessed with a pinhole to give an estimate of the final corrected vision if the patient's glasses are not available. The corneal curvature should be examined by **keratometry**, which is a measure of the refractive power of areas of the cornea, and by **corneal topography**, which is a measure of the steepness of various areas of the cornea; both of these are usually automated.

Management

Treatment should only be undertaken if it is necessary, e.g. if the patient is symptomatic or visual correction is required for legal or employment reasons. The most common form of correction is with cylindrical optical spectacle correction.

Soft contact lenses are useful but are more costly as they have to be specially made to enable them to stay in the correct position for corneal curvature. Hard contact lenses alter the shape of the cornea, thus correcting mild astigmatism.

Corneal laser refractive surgery is increasingly popular. It can be used to correct mild to moderate astigmatism.

Prognosis

The prognosis is generally very good for the correction of astigmatism.

4.5 Presbyopia

Presbyopia is the reduction in accommodative ability with age.

Epidemiology

Loss of **accommodation**, the change in the eye's focus for near objects, is remarkably consistent throughout all populations and between the sexes. The amount of possible accommodation gradually declines with time, reaching almost zero by the age of 50 (**Figure 4.4**).

Pathogenesis

Presbyopia is part of the normal ageing of the lens and its capsule, ciliary body and zonular fibres. With time, the lens and capsule become less elastic and hence less able to become thicker to assist in accommodation. The elastic ability almost halves between the ages of 20 and 40. The ciliary body has a smaller effect and, in later years, is less able to contract and hence enable accommodation. The change in the zonular fibre

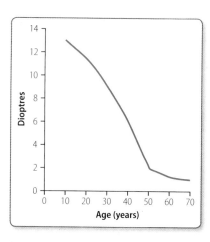

Figure 4.4 The decline in accommodation with age

attachment on the lens capsule means that accommodation may be more difficult.

Clinical features

The clinical features of presbyopia include:

· patients being older than 40
· difficulty with near work
· tiredness/strain especially when reading

Diagnostic criteria

Presbyopia is diagnosed when patients have normal distance vision but reduced near vision. The near vision can be corrected by the addition of convergent (+) lenses.

Clinical insight

Some myopes may never be affected as reading distance will focus light perfectly on the back of the eye without refractive correction.

Investigations

Accommodation should be measured objectively by using a ruler. Letters can be placed on the end of the ruler and the ruler gradually moved towards the patient. When the patient indicates that the letters are blurred, the distance between the patient and the ruler should be noted. The near-point (or RAF) rule is a device used to measure the near points of accommodation and convergence.

Differential diagnosis

Occasionally, a failure of accommodation mimics presbyopia. This is differentiated by other ocular signs, such as a dilated pupil, as in Adie's pupil (tonic dilated pupil), and third nerve (oculomotor nerve) palsy. A history of sudden onset can also indicate failure of accommodation.

Management

Symptoms can be corrected by convergent (+) lensed spectacles that compensate for the accommodative loss. If there are no other refractive abnormalities, plain reading spectacles may be appropriate. Otherwise, the choice between bifocal and varifocal lenses can be discussed with the patient. Although there is no treatment to cure or prevent presbyopia, recent developments in accommodating intraocular lens technology enable recovery of some accommodative ability.

Prognosis

Presbyopia is easily treated with spectacle correction.

Orbital diseases increase the volume of the orbital contents, pushing the globe forward (**proptosis**) and compressing the orbital contents such as the optic nerve. Consequently, all orbital diseases can be potentially severe and sight threatening. Orbital disease occurs relatively infrequently, but it is important to consider the structures surrounding the orbit both as potential sources of orbital disease, such as the **sinuses** (mucous lined air spaces in the skull), and as potential areas for disease spread, such as the brain.

Anatomy

The orbit is a cone-shaped, bone-lined compartment that contains the globe and the extraocular muscles (**Figure 5.1**). Anteriorly, it is separated from the outer eyelids by the **orbital septum** (a fibrous layer enabling the attachment of the lid muscles), and is surrounded medially, inferiorly and superiorly by the sinuses. Apertures allow sensory (especially optic and nasociliary) and motor (third, fourth and sixth cranial) nerves to communicate with the orbital structures.

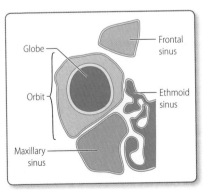

Figure 5.1 The orbit in coronal section and the sinuses surrounding the orbit.

Unlike the eye, no orbital structures can be directly visualised, and the presence of orbital disease has to be inferred by the presence of a change in position of the globe, a restriction of eye movements or a reduction in visual function.

5.1 Clinical scenario

Rapid lid swelling

Presentation

An 8-year-old girl presents to the emergency department with rapid swelling of the right lid.

Diagnostic approach

The first aim is to try to exclude causes that require urgent treatment, e.g. orbital cellulitis or thyroid eye disease. Orbital cellulitis is a rapid-onset unilateral inflammation of the orbit and lid. Thyroid eye disease is usually a chronic-onset, asymmetric, but bilateral, eye disease.

> ### Guiding principle
>
> Lid swelling can be a sign of diseases that can cause blindness and, rarely, death.

Diagnostic clues in the history This patient describes unilateral and rapid-onset swelling. This would exclude thyroid eye disease but not orbital cellulitis. Other differential diagnoses in this condition include orbital inflammatory disease and preseptal cellulitis. Orbital inflammatory disease is rare and has signs similar to orbital cellulitis. Therefore, the next stage is to ask about the origin of the condition and any associated symptoms. See **Table 5.1** for a summary of the causes of lid swelling.

Further history

The lid swelling has occurred over the last day with redness and is tender to touch. The problem affects the upper and lower lids on one eye. The child has recently had an illness and has had a runny nose and complained of a sore forehead and cheeks.

Previous medical history The patient's immunisations are up to date and her development is normal.

	Rapid onset	Chronic onset
Localised	**Chalazion:** lid lump, usually tender when active Hordeolum: localised tender swelling usually most prominent at the lid margin	**Tumour:** various different forms, most commonly at the lower lid margin. Possible history of sun exposure
Diffuse	**Preseptal cellulitis:** warm, red, and tender, usually with an instigating factor **Orbital cellulitis:** generalised swelling of upper and lower lids; in late stages, reduced vision and double vision Inflammatory orbital disease: symptoms similar to orbital cellulitis **Severe conjunctivitis:** possible preceding viral illness with red and watery eyes	**Thyroid eye disease:** bilateral chronic redness of eyes. In later stages, double vision and 'staring eyes' **Nephrotic syndrome:** bilateral lid swelling, especially on lying down; marked swelling of ankles

Table 5.1   Lid swelling: causes and symptoms

Diagnostic approach

The further history does not indicate any cause for preseptal cellulitis, which would normally have an external instigating factor such as a skin break or eyelid infection. However, orbital cellulitis is much more likely with a history of recent illness and soreness of the sinuses.

Examination

The patient looks unwell and her temperature is 39.4°C.

Ophthalmic examination There is obvious lid swelling and, when the lid is lifted, the eye appears red. See **Table 5.2** for a summary of the remaining clinical examination.

Diagnostic approach

The patient appears to have signs of orbital cellulitis (reduced vision, relative afferent pupil defect, reduced colour vision, injected conjunctiva and reduced ocular motility). This is an

	Right eye	Left eye
6/60	**Visual acuity (with glasses)**	6/6
Normal direct and consensual reflex, but right RAPD	**Pupil**	Normal direct and consensual reflex and no RAPD
Clear	**Cornea**	Clear
Clear	**Anterior chamber**	Clear
Clear	**Lens**	Clear
Clear	**Vitreous**	Clear
Clear view of fundus	**Fundus**	Clear view of fundus
Disc vessels appear tortuous and congested	**Disc**	Normal vessels and disc
Reduced	**Ishihara test**	Normal
The eye is displaced laterally and there is a restriction of movement in abduction and adduction	**Ocular motility**	Full range of movement

RAPD, relative afferent pupil defect.

Table 5.2 Ophthalmic examination: results for a patient who presented with lid swelling

ocular and systemic emergency and requires urgent notification to paediatric and ENT colleagues. The patient should be kept nil by mouth initially and a CT scan organised, as she may have a subperiosteal abscess requiring drainage. In the interim period, nasal decongestants and intravenous antibiotics can be instituted.

5.2 Preseptal cellulitis and orbital cellulitis

The orbital septum is a fibrous band of tissue that extends from the orbital rim to the tarsal plate and that separates the anterior in front from the orbit behind. Preseptal cellulitis is the term given to infection of the soft tissues anterior to the septum. Infection of the tissues posterior to the orbital septum is termed orbital cellulitis. Differentiating the two conditions is crucial as orbital cellulitis is potentially sight and life threatening. The management of orbital cellulitis demands close liaison between ophthalmologists and their ENT colleagues to ensure an optimum outcome.

Epidemiology
Of those patients affected with orbital cellulitis, 80% are children under the age of 10 years.

Causes
Preseptal cellulitis is usually associated with an obvious antecedent cause such as a tarsal cyst or injury. Orbital cellulitis almost always results from the spread of infection from the adjacent paranasal sinuses.

Pathogenesis
The paranasal sinuses are symmetrical, paired, mucosa-lined spaces which surround the orbits. They communicate with the nasal space via small openings (ostea). Blockage of the ostea results in a build-up of mucus that can easily become infected, effectively turning the sinus into an abscess.

As the bony walls of the sinuses are thin and have small perforations for communicating vessels, any infection can directly spread into the orbit. The resulting soft-tissue swelling can frequently cause marked compression of the contents, including the optic nerve. Spread of infection via the orbital veins can result in life-threatening complications, such as cavernous sinus thrombosis and cerebral abscess.

The most common organisms isolated from cases of preseptal cellulitis are *Staphylococcus aureus*, *Staphylococcus epidermidis* and *Streptococcus pyogenes*.

Clinical features

Symptoms include swelling and redness of the lids without proptosis or reduced eye movements (**Figure 5.1**) both in preseptal cellulitis and in the early stages of orbital cellulitis. Key signs of orbital disease include:

- proptosis
- reduced eye movements
- optic neuropathy

Figure 5.2 shows reddened swelling of both upper and lower lids, ptosis and proptosis.

> ### Clinical insight
>
> It can be difficult to differentiate orbital from preseptal cellulitis. Erring on the side of caution, assume it is orbital unless there are definite signs of eyelid trauma, a cyst or infection.

Diagnostic criteria

The staging of preseptal/ orbital cellulitis is clinical (**Table 5.3**).

Investigations

Most physicians will scan patients with suspected orbital cellulitis to confirm the presence of pan-sinusitis and to identify any subperiosteal abscess. Investigations should include a systemic work-up with full blood count and blood cultures.

> ### Clinical insight
>
> If proptosis is non-axial (in addition to the eye being displaced outwards it is also displaced laterally/inferiorly/superiorly), it will signify the development of a subperiosteal abscess. This will require immediate drainage, which is usually performed by ENT colleagues; however, if the patient is young and is not showing signs of proptosis and optic nerve compression, it is acceptable to wait 2 days for IV antibiotics to work provided the vision is monitored regularly.

Differential diagnosis

The differential diagnoses include:

- non-specific orbital inflammatory disease
- dermoid cysts or a choristoma [congenital lesions representing normal tissue(s) in an abnormal location]; occasionally, these leak, inciting a brisk inflammatory reaction

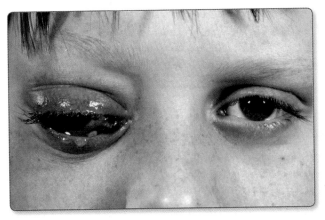

Figure 5.2 Orbital cellulitis.

Stage	Description
1	Preseptal cellulitis
2	Orbital cellulitis
3	Subperiosteal abscess
4	Orbital abscess
5	Cavernous sinus thrombosis

Table 5.3 Classification of orbital cellulitis

Management

Preseptal cellulitis is treated with:
- oral antibiotics initially

Orbital cellulitis is treated with:
- intravenous broad-spectrum antibiotics if patients have, or are suspected of having, orbital cellulitis; patients should be admitted for frequent clinical assessment and treatment
- nasal decongestants

Drainage of subperiosteal abscess, if identified, should be carried out by ENT colleagues.

Prognosis

Preseptal cellulitis almost never results in long-term complications. Orbital cellulitis is a medical emergency, with a risk of permanent loss of vision and even death from cerebral spread of infection.

5.3 Thyroid orbitopathy

Thyroid orbitopathy (TO) is a chronic, self-limiting, autoimmune inflammatory condition that is usually associated with abnormal thyroid function, most commonly Graves disease. Usually, the signs of orbital inflammation will coexist with the systemic effects of a thyroid hormonal imbalance. Treatment often requires a multidisciplinary approach, which includes an ophthalmologist, endocrinologist and ENT/ophthalmic orbital surgeon.

Epidemiology

Between one quarter and one half of patients with **Graves disease** (an autoimmune thyroid disease) have some form of TO. The disease is five times more common among women than men, and peaks in incidence during the 5th and 7th decades.

Causes

TO is most commonly linked with hyperthyroidism, usually Graves disease; however, 15% of cases of TO are associated with primary hypothyroidism. Other, less common, thyroid conditions can have similar manifestations, including Hashimoto disease, thyroid carcinoma and primary hyperthyroidism. Note that patients with normal thyroid levels can develop TO.

Clinical insight

Smoking has been found to result in an increased incidence and severity of thyroid eye disease, and patients with thyroid orbitopathy should be counselled to cease smoking.

Pathogenesis

TO results from abnormal autoimmune activation of cells normally resident in the orbit. Circulating thyroid receptor antibodies are thought to activate resident fibroblasts, which, in turn, release chemokines. The chemokines attract T-helper cells. Activated T-helper cells then release cytokines that induce adipogenesis, fibroblast proliferation, glycosaminoglycan formation and B-cell activation, which causes an exponential increase in effect. This inflammatory reaction leads to an increase in intraorbital volume and fibrosis of extraocular muscles.

Clinical features

The symptoms of TO include:
- chronic redness of the eye
- corneal irritation
- double vision
- others noting staring eyes

The signs include:

Clinical insight

Thyroid orbitopathy is frequently asymmetrical, but usually affects both eyes eventually.

- proptosis (when combined with thyroid abnormality, this is often called exophthalmos) in one quarter of patients (**Figure 5.3**)
- extraocular muscle restriction in one quarter of patients; this most commonly involves inferior rectus and medial rectus fibrosis, which leads to restriction of movement in the opposite direction to muscle action

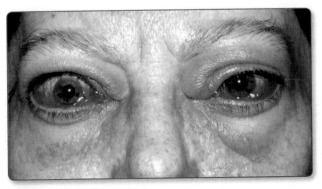

Figure 5.3 Active thyroid orbitopathy.

Diagnostic criteria

Various different diagnostic and monitoring criteria have been developed. A commonly used scoring system to monitor disease severity is shown in **Table 5.4**.

Investigations

The following investigations should be carried out:

- blood tests, including thyrotrophin receptor antibodies and generalised thyroid function tests
- in suspected optic nerve compression, CT or MRI

Clinical insight

Severe thyroid eye disease should be treated as an ophthalmic emergency, with regular monitoring of vision, colour vision, corneal surface, proptosis, ocular movements and optic nerve appearance. Loss of vision, which is occasionally permanent, can ensue by two main mechanisms. First, the exophthalmos can lead to corneal exposure, drying the corneal epithelium. Second, the increased volume of the orbital contents can cause increased pressure on the optic nerve, resulting in optic neuropathy and eventual atrophy. In both cases, patients complain of worsening vision.

Symptom or sign	Score 1 mark for each feature present: Total = 10
Chemosis	
Conjunctival injection	
Lid oedema	
Pain at rest	
Pain on movement	
Chemosis of lids	
Chemosis of conjunctiva	
Increased proptosis ≥2 mm	
Decrease in eye movement by ≥5°	
Decrease in visual acuity by one Snellen line or more	

Table 5.4 Clinical activity score for thyroid eye disease. Modified from Mourits et al., Clinical Endocrinology 1997;47:9-14. Ocular Surface 2007;5:163–78

Differential diagnosis

The differential diagnoses include:

- *conjunctivitis*: causes discharge that resolves with time or treatment
- *orbital tumour*: this is usually unilateral
- *caroticocavernous fistula*: if there is a previous history of trauma

Management

Active disease should be treated with immunosuppression: a course of intravenous corticosteroid with or without low-dose orbital radiation to try to modify the clinical course of the disease. Surgery should be reserved for inactive disease or only for sight-threatening active disease. Surgery should be carried out in a stepwise fashion – orbital decompression before squint surgery followed by eyelid surgery – although not all patients will require all three surgical steps.

Prognosis

TO usually resolves within 24 months of onset. The prognosis is very good for the majority of patients as they have only mild symptoms. However, those diagnosed late and those who are older, male or have highly active disease still have a risk of loss of vision. Careful monitoring, aggressive treatment of activity and stepwise correction after disease cessation usually lead to a good final outcome.

Eyelid and lacrimal apparatus

Eyelid abnormalities and excessive tearing often result in patients presenting to both primary and secondary care. The eyelids have specialised glands that commonly get blocked or infected. In addition, ageing results in increased eyelid structural problems because of greater laxity of tissues and their attachments.

Although they do not jeopardise vision, in the majority of cases these conditions result in marked morbidity caused by alteration of the normal corneal tear film and corneal epithelial changes.

Anatomy and physiology

The eyelids are specialised mucous membrane- and skin-lined muscular curtains that resurface the eye with tears, which are principally produced by the lacrimal gland. They contain canaliculi that drain the tears into the lacrimal sac, and then into the nose via the nasolacrimal sac (**Figure 2.7**).

The upper lid is held open principally by the **levator palpebrae superioris muscle**; the **Müller muscle** (superior tarsal muscle) contributes to the resting eyelid height by only 1–2 mm. Lid malpositions include turning in (**entropion**), turning out (**ectropion**), and lid height abnormalities.

The skin of the eyelids is extremely thin and is loosely bound to the underlying orbicularis muscle, allowing for a greater range of movement (**Figure 6.1**). Failure of the lids to close (**lagophthalmos**) will quickly be complicated by corneal drying and ulceration.

6.1 Clinical scenarios

Watery eye

Presentation

A 60-year-old woman presents to the outpatient department complaining of a 3-month history of a watery right eye.

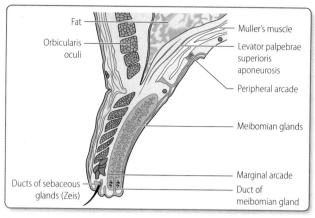

Figure 6.1 Cross-section of the eyelid.

Diagnostic approach

Epiphora (wateriness) occurs secondary to either increased tear production or reduced tear drainage (**Table 6.1**). In conditions secondary to increased tear production, the patient's epiphora will usually be associated with other symptoms, such as foreign body sensation, itch or photophobia. In patients with unilateral disease, the appearance of the unaffected and affected sides should be directly compared, looking for anatomical differences to explain the epiphora.

Further history

The patient's epiphora is not associated with any other symptoms. There is no prior history of painful red swelling in the medial canthal area.

Previous medical history The patient is not atopic (asthma/eczema/hayfever); however, she does have hypertension.

Previous ocular history The patient wears reading glasses.

Medications The patient takes bendroflumethiazide for her hypertension.

Increased tear production	Decreased tear drainage
Corneal irritation, e.g. foreign body, trichiasis	Ectropion
Conjunctival disease, e.g. conjunctivitis	Lid laxity
Lid disease, e.g. blepharitis	Facial nerve palsy
Reduced tear film quality	Stenosis of the puncta, canaliculus or nasolacrimal duct

Table 6.1 Common causes of watery eye

Diagnostic approach
Examination
The patient is generally well with no obvious neurological deficit of the cranial nerves.

Ophthalmic examination For a summary of the ophthalmic examination, see **Table 6.2**.

Diagnostic approach
As there is no significant difference in the apposition of the lids to the globe, size of the puncta or quality of the blink, logically the explanation is a difference between the lacrimal outflow passages, which are explored with a diagnostic sac wash-out (SWO), a procedure used to check the patency of tear outflow.

Investigations There is regurgitation of fluid via both the lower and upper puncta on SWO and an impression of a 'hard stop' (lacrimal bone), i.e. the site of the obstruction is below the lacrimal sac, when the cannula is advanced towards the lacrimal sac.

The SWO confirms the presence of a blocked nasolacrimal duct.

Lid lumps
Presentation
A 65-year-old man presents to his GP's surgery with a 3-month history of a slowly increasing left lower lid lump.

	Right eye		Left eye
	6/6	**Visual acuity**	6/6
	No signs of blepharitis Normal lid position, i.e. no ectropion/entropion or trichiasis Upper and lower puncta are both present and open Normal symmetrical blink observed No swelling observed in the lacrimal sac area and no regurgitation of mucus or pus when pressure is applied to the lacrimal sac area No signs of inflammation of the tarsal conjunctiva	**Lid**	No signs of blepharitis No entropion/ectropion Upper and lower puncta are both present and open Normal symmetrical blink observed No swelling observed in the lacrimal sac area and no regurgitation of mucus or pus when pressure is applied to the lacrimal sac area No signs of inflammation of the tarsal conjunctiva
	No foreign bodies No fluorescein uptake Normal tear film break-up	**Cornea**	No foreign bodies No fluorescein uptake Normal tear film break-up
	White	**Conjunctiva**	White

Table 6.2 Ophthalmic examination: results for a patient who presented with watery eye

Diagnostic approach

Lumps are a common reason for ophthalmic referral (for causes of lid lumps, see **Table 6.3**). The lids are composed of the **anterior lamella**, which consists of skin (containing various adnexal structures) and the orbicularis muscle, and the **posterior lamella**, which is lined by conjunctiva and contains the **tarsal plate** – the tough margin of the lids in which the **tarsal glands** (**meibomian glands**) are located. It is therefore diagnostically useful to try to ascertain which lamella the mass is arising from.

Further history

The patient does not have any pain or tenderness.

Lid lump	Characteristic features
Cyst of Moll (sudoriferous cyst)	Clear fluid-filled cyst, translucent and transilluminates
Cyst of Zeis (sebaceous cyst of lid margin)	Round white lump filled with oily secretions
External hordeolum (stye)	Tender, red abscess around a lash follicle
Chalazion (meibomian cyst)	Small pea-sized lump arising from the tarsal plate. In the acute phase, it will be tender and red
Sebaceous cyst	Opaque cyst filled with yellow material. The cyst has a definite punctum
Seborrhoeic keratoses	Flattish, plaque-like greasy lesions
Basal cell carcinoma	Most commonly nodular with rolled, pearly edges, telangiectasia and sometimes with a central ulcer
Squamous cell carcinoma	Similar to basal cell carcinoma but usually with excess keratinisation and may ulcerate

Table 6.3 Common lid lumps

Previous medical history The patient has previously had a cancerous skin lesion removed from his face.

Examination

Ophthalmic examination Examination reveals a raised, pearly-edged lump on the right lower lid with an ulcerated crater (**Figure 6.2**). There is a focal loss of lashes around the lesion. There is no inflammation present on the tarsal plate in the same area as the lesion. There are no signs of **blepharitis** (lid inflammation) or of generalised skin disease. There are a few areas of reddened scaly plaques on the patient's face.

Diagnostic approach

The lack of preceding tenderness or pain in the history and

the absence of redness of the tarsal plate indicate a malignant process rather than an inflammatory one. Often, patients with recurrent chalazia will have local risk factors such as blepharitis or specific dermatological risk factors such as rosacea. This patient has cutaneous signs of solar damage (**actinic keratoses**) and a history of having a previous skin malignancy. The hallmark of malignancy is invasion of surrounding tissues and the destruction of normal structures – in this case the lash follicles, hence the loss of eyelashes.

Investigations Definitive diagnosis is made by biopsy, preferably excisional, if the diagnosis is not in doubt; however, the description points to a **basal cell carcinoma**, a malignant but slow-spreading cancer of the epithelium.

6.2 Entropion

Entropion is an in-turning or inversion of the eyelid margin.

Epidemiology

Entropion accounts for approximately 10% of oculoplastic referrals. There is an ethnic variation in incidence, with Asian

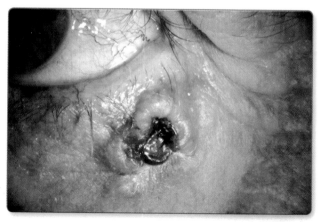

Figure 6.2 Patient presenting with a lid lesion.

populations being affected more frequently than others. In Western countries, the incidence of entropion increases with age and most commonly affects the lower lid.

Causes

For the causes of entropion, see **Table 6.4**.

Pathogenesis

Entropion effectively results from forces that predispose the anterior lamella to override the posterior lamella. The vertical height of the tarsus of the upper lid is three times greater than that of the lower lid; hence, the upper lid is intrinsically more stable, and upper lid entropion is always secondary to cicatricial causes.

> ## Clinical insight
>
> A good analogy for the lids is to think of them as a tennis court net. In order for the lid to retain good position, it has to be under a degree of tension (canthal tendons) and be attached to the floor (inferior retractor).

Clinical features

Patients with entropion complain of irritable red eyes that tear regularly and are associated with a foreign body sensation. It is important to ask for a history of mouth or skin ulceration, which would suggest an underlying systemic cicatrising disease.

Examination includes looking for signs of conjunctival scarring, which is seen as a white band, and corneal decompensation from in-turning lashes (**Figure 6.3**). The laxity of the tendons

Type	Cause
Involutional	Laxity of canthal ligaments The preseptal overriding the pretarsal orbicularis Retractor dehiscence
Cicatricial	Contraction of the posterior lamella caused by infection (trachoma), injury (chemical burn) or autoimmune disease (ocular cicatricial pemphigoid)
Spastic	Overaction of orbicularis secondary to ocular surface irritation

Table 6.4 Causes of entropion

can be measured by horizontal stretch tests and a snap test, in which the lid is pulled away from the face and released.

Differential diagnosis

Entropion is sometimes confused with other conditions that lead to lashes in-turning. These include:

- *trichiasis*, with lashes growing inwards
- *distichiasis*, in which a row of extra lashes is found near the eyelid margin
- *epiblepharon*, in which an extra fold of skin pushes lashes inwards

> **Clinical insight**
>
> Conjunctival scarring may be a sign of cicatricial disease such as pemphigoid, which leads to bilateral and systemic disease.

Management

Management varies with the cause and severity of entropion:

- *Involutional* (degenerative). This should be treated surgically by everting sutures to turn the lid outwards, preventing overriding of the orbicularis. Four or five 4/0 Vicryl Rapide

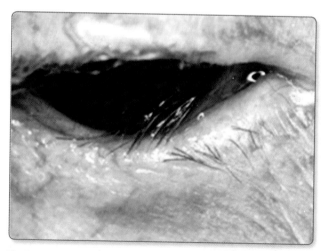

Figure 6.3 Entropion with lashes causing corneal abrasion.

(Ethicon) sutures are ideal for this purpose and can be placed at the first consultation. However, if there is recurrence, permanent resolution is unlikely without some form of lid shortening

- *Cicatricial* (scarring related). Surgery requires division of the scarring band and lengthening of the posterior lamella. The posterior lamella can be extended by inserting graft material from the buccal mucosa, hard palate or ear cartilage

Prognosis

Involutional entropion corrected by everting sutures results in an 85% chance of the patient remaining entropion free for the next 4 years. Cicatricial entropion is usually secondary to autoimmune disease, such as ocular cicatricial pemphigoid, which is often progressive despite systemic immunosuppression with up to one third of these patients eventually being registered blind.

6.3 Ectropion

Ectropion is an out-turning or eversion of the eyelid margin.

Epidemiology

Ectropion accounts for approximately 10% of oculoplastic referrals.

Causes

For the causes of ectropion, see **Table 6.5**.

Pathogenesis

Ectropion shares many of the same causatory factors as entropion and results from forces that predispose the posterior lamella to override the anterior lamella (**Table 6.3**).

Clinical features

Patients with ectropion complain of the abnormal appearance of the lid; in addition, the tarsal conjunctiva of the everted lid becomes inflamed, which is often associated with wateriness

Type	Cause
Involutional	Laxity of canthal ligaments Retractor dehiscence
Cicatricial	Skin scarring caused by injury (burns), excessive skin removal (injudicious surgery) or chronic inflammation (eczema)
Paralytic	Lower motor seventh nerve palsy, e.g. Bell's palsy (idiopathic lower motor neurone CN VII palsy) acoustic neuroma Upper motor seventh nerve, e.g. secondary to stroke
Mechanical	Tumour, e.g. basal cell carcinoma, sebaceous cell carcinoma Infection/inflammation, e.g. chalazion

Table 6.5 Causes of ectropion

and discharge. Examination will reveal an everted lid (**Figure 6.4**).

Note should be made of any tightness of the skin; ectropion is often secondary to eczema, is occasionally due to scarring and, rarely, is due to a cicatrising skin cancer such as basal cell carcinoma. Laxity of the lid should be assessed as described above, with particular attention being paid to orbicularis function to detect signs of facial nerve palsy. This can be done by testing the patient's ability to resist forcible opening of the closed eyelids.

Differential diagnosis

A chalazion can be associated with an inflamed lid margin, but the lid margin will be in a normal position.

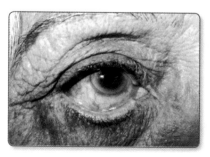

Figure 6.4 Ectropion.

Management

Management varies with the cause and severity of ectropion:

- *Involutional*. This should be treated surgically by horizontal lid shortening, usually combined with reinsertion of the lower lid retractors via a conjunctival approach. Topical corticosteroid ointment should be prescribed for the 4 weeks preceding the operation to reduce tarsal conjunctival inflammation
- *Cicatricial*. Surgery requires division of any skin scarring and then lengthening of the anterior lamella by the addition of new skin as grafts or flaps. Donor tissue sites include the upper eyelids, upper arm and posterior auricular skin
- *Paralytic*. Orbicularis tone can sometimes be restored following cross-facial nerve grafting, which is a complicated surgical procedure usually reserved for younger patients with significant loss of facial nerve function. Much more commonly, the lids are simply tightened with horizontal lid shortening, and rarely with fascial slings
- *Mechanical*. This includes surgical excision of the lesion

Prognosis

The prognosis is generally very good for ectropion following repair; however, as with all involutional pathology, recurrences are common.

6.4 Ptosis

Ptosis is the name given to a drooping upper eyelid.

Epidemiology

Ptosis constitutes 30% of all oculoplastic referrals; this is partly because of an increasingly elderly population, but also because of greater awareness of cosmetic correction.

Causes

The most common cause is involutional ptosis (for a summary of causes, see **Table 6.6**).

Pathogenesis

It is helpful to review the anatomy of the eyelid to help understand the pathogenesis of ptosis (see Anatomy and physiology). Stretching or dehiscence of the levator palpebrae superioris aponeurosis is the most common cause of ptosis in the elderly (**Figure 6.5**). Weakness of the levator muscle, because of either congenital maldevelopment (dystrophy) or acquired myopathic causes or impairment of the third cranial nerve supply to the levator, will also result in ptosis.

The Müller muscle is supplied by the sympathetic chain; impairment of sympathetic innervation is often termed Horner syndrome (oculosympathetic palsy) and usually leads to a ptosis of only 1–2 mm.

Clinical features

Particular attention should be paid to:

- measuring the levator function with the excursion of the lid in extreme downgaze to extreme upgaze; this is normally more than 12 mm
- the height of the lid crease should be measured; this is normally 6 mm in men and 8 mm in women
- a high or absent lid crease is the hallmark of an aponeurotic ptosis (**Figure 6.5**)

Type	Cause
Neurogenic	Third nerve palsy
	Horner syndrome (oculosympathetic palsy)
Aponeurotic	Involutional dehiscence/detachment of levator
	Traumatic dehiscence/detachment of levator
Myogenic	Myasthenia gravis
	Myotonic dystrophies
	Chronic progressive external ophthalmoplegia
	Congenital dystrophic levator malformation
Mechanical	Tumour
	Enlarged lacrimal gland

Table 6.6 Causes of ptosis

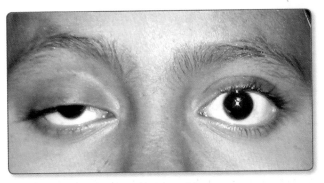

Figure 6.5 Aponeurotic ptosis with an absent lid crease.

- the presence of anisocoria (unequal pupil sizes) is consistent with a neurogenic cause

Next, the extraocular movements should be assessed. A gaze palsy, if associated with reduced levator function, indicates a myogenic cause. The superior fornix should be inspected and palpated for any masses (most commonly lymphoma), which can be associated with a mechanical ptosis.

Investigations

Investigations are not usually warranted in aponeurotic ptosis, but they are usually performed for other causes of ptosis. Acquired Horner syndrome requires a chest radiograph to exclude apical lung tumour. If myasthenia is suspected, an ice pack test can be performed and blood markers of myasthenia can be assessed (see Chapter 13). Myogenic causes can sometimes be diagnosed by muscle biopsy.

Clinical insight

A smaller pupil on the ptotic side indicates Horner syndrome; a larger pupil, particularly if associated with reduced eye movements, indicates third nerve palsy.

Differential diagnosis

A commonly encountered cause of pseudoptosis is derma-tochalasis (i.e. excessive upper lid skin that hangs over the lids in a fold and mimics the presence of ptosis). Other causes include enophthalmos, microphthalmia or hypotropia of the ipsilateral side and lid retraction or proptosis of the contralateral side.

Management

If the underlying cause cannot be rectified, surgery is the mainstay of treatment. The type of surgery depends on the levator function:

- >5 mm – the levator aponeurosis/muscle is shortened/advanced
- <5 mm – a brow suspension is performed, which involves surgically connecting the frontalis muscle/tendon to the eyelid

Surgery is avoided in myogenic causes. In myasthenia, oral pyridostigmine can be tried to maximise the levator muscle function. Ptosis props can be used but are not especially effective.

Prognosis

The prognosis in aponeurotic ptosis is good. However, in patients with myogenic ptosis it can be difficult to achieve sufficient lid opening to improve vision without preventing the lid from closing properly, which can result in corneal ulceration.

6.5 Blepharitis

Blepharitis is the common name for a range of eyelid inflammations. It is usually differentiated anatomically into anterior, involving the lashes, and posterior, involving the meibomian glands.

Epidemiology

Blepharitis is a common disorder and is often referred for ophthalmic opinion.

Causes

Blepharitis may occur without any obvious cause. Specific causes include rosacea, allergy, bacterial infection including *Staphylococcus*, viral infection including herpes and molluscum, fungal infection including seborrhoeic dermatitis, and parasitic infection with demodex.

Pathogenesis

Most commonly, this results from a build-up of bacteria on either the lash follicles or meibomian orifices. The subsequent immune response causes collateral damage and inflammation, as does release of bacterial toxins. Anteriorly, this results in an inflammatory response on the skin surrounding the lashes. Posteriorly, gland function can be disrupted with a secondary dry eye due to tear film instability.

Clinical features

Patients with blepharitis present with a burning sensation, watering from the eyes and occasionally foreign body sensation if the cornea is involved. Examination reveals a red, inflamed eyelid (**Figure 6.6**). Occasionally, corneal staining may be seen with fluorescein dye. It is useful to exclude other specific causes of blepharitis by examining for rosacea or other signs of viral and fungal infection on the face.

Investigations

For simple blepharitis no further investigation is required. However, if chronic, a swab can be taken for resistant bacteria.

Differential diagnosis

Lid swelling can sometimes be mistaken for:

- early preseptal cellulitis or other inflammatory/infectious causes, including chalazion or hordeolum; usually, there is an element of pain in these conditions
- early morphoeic basal cell carcinoma or sebaceous cell carcinoma; these are, however, unilateral and are associated

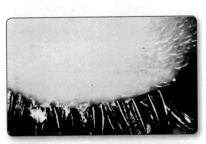

Figure 6.6 Blepharitis.

with loss of normal lid architecture, most often observed as loss of lashes

Management

If the onset is relatively acute, it is important to exclude the use of topical agents (including mascara and eye drops) that can cause local allergic reactions. Treatment consists of local measures that help to reduce the bacterial load by removing the crusts that can build up on the lash roots and the use of topical chloramphenicol ointment.

To assist meibomian gland function, the glands can be expressed with a warm compress. If, despite these measures, the lid margins remain inflamed, a corticosteroid ointment can be used sparingly. Persistent inflammation of the meibomian glands can often respond to a short, 2- to 3-week course of oral tetracyclines (e.g. doxycycline 50 mg per day). Tear supplements can be given if there is a poor tear film or the cornea is involved.

Prognosis

The prognosis is good, but patients should be counselled that, in the vast majority of cases, blepharitis cannot be completely cured. However, the symptoms can be controlled if the patient complies with the treatment.

6.6 Chalazion

Chalazion is commonly known as a meibomian or tarsal cyst and results from a localised inflammation of the meibomian gland and is often associated with blepharitis (see above).

Epidemiology

These are common infections and inflammations. Chalazia can occur in children as well as in adults, but are more common in adults.

Causes

Recurrent chalazia are likely to be associated with blepharitis.

Pathogenesis

The initiating factor in chalazia is a blockage or reduced flow of secretions at or before the duct opening. This may be secondary to infection or inflammation of the ducts or due to thick secretions. In the chalazion, the build-up of secretions leads to gland rupture, causing a granulomatous inflammatory reaction in the surrounding tissues. The most common infective cause is *Staphylococcus aureus*.

Clinical features

Acutely, patients complain of a red, painful swollen eyelid (**Figure 6.7**). Chalazia that do not resolve by 6 weeks are likely to persist with a chronically inflamed lid mass that characteristically is associated with a focal area of redness on the tarsal plate but occasionally can be more obvious on the skin side. Examination may also reveal predisposing causes such as rosacea or blepharitis.

Investigations

If the chalazion has an atypical appearance or fails to respond to treatment, an appropriate biopsy should be undertaken to establish the diagnosis.

Differential diagnosis

The differential diagnoses include:
- *preseptal cellulitis*: erythema and tenderness spreads beyond a focal area

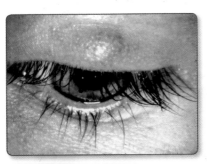

Figure 6.7 A chalazion (meibomian cyst).

- *basal cell carcinoma*: usually non-tender; loss of lashes may occur
- *sebaceous cell carcinoma*: persistent chalazion-type lesions

Management

Treatment is targeted at restoring the flow of oils from the blocked meibomian gland orifice(s). In the acute stage, this process may be expedited by opening the gland orifices with the aid of regular warm compresses followed by digital compression of the affected lid margin. Inflammation of the lid margins/gland orifices can be lessened by the use of topical corticosteroid ointment. Chronic (>6 weeks) chalazia can be treated by incision and curettage if a cyst is palpable.

Systemic antibiotic treatment is warranted only if the chalazion becomes infected and preseptal cellulitis develops.

> **Clinical insight**
>
> Counselling for continued lid hygiene is required even after recovery to prevent recurrence.

Prognosis

Prognosis is good for chalazia, with complete recovery the norm.

6.7 Eyelid malignancies

Only 20% of eyelid tumours are malignant. There are several different types of eyelid malignancy. The key features of malignant eyelid lesions in general and the clinical features of the types of carcinoma specifically are described here.

Epidemiology

Malignant eyelid lesions are relatively common and account for approximately 16 cases per 100,000 of the population. Basal cell carcinoma (BCC) constitutes 90–95% of eyelid malignancies, with squamous cell carcinoma (SCC) constituting another 5–10% of cases. Most commonly, this occurs in middle-aged to elderly fair-skinned people. Eyelid tumours are slightly more common in men than in women. Sebaceous cell carcinomas and Merkel cell tumours (primary neuroendocrine carcinomas) are rare but clinically important because of the relatively high rate of metastatic spread. **Table 6.7** summarises premalignant and malignant eyelid tumours.

Causes

The causes of eyelid malignancies include:

- ultraviolet sun exposure
- conversion of premalignant lesions
- immunosuppression
- Gorlin syndrome (naevoid BCC syndrome) – an autosomal dominant condition predisposing patients to multiple BCCs
- xeroderma pigmentosum – a DNA mismatch repair defect predisposing patients to SCC

Pathogenesis

The main pathogenetic pathway of malignancy is by direct DNA damage from radiation, which is thought to cause a mutation of tumour suppressor genes. The second pathogenetic pathway is ultraviolet light, which suppresses the dermal cellular immune response, allowing the tumour to grow unchallenged.

Clinical features

Table 6.8 summarises the clinical features of various different types of tumour. Examples of BCC and SCC are shown in **Figure 6.8**.

Premalignant eyelid lesions	Malignant eyelid tumours
Actinic keratosis	Basal cell carcinoma (**Figure 6.8a**)
Bowen disease (squamous cell carcinoma in situ)	Squamous cell carcinoma (**Figure 6.8b**)
Keratoacanthoma	Malignant melanoma
	Sebaceous cell carcinoma
	Merkel cell tumour (primary neuroendocrine carcinoma)

Table 6.7 Types of premalignant and malignant eyelid tumours

Malignancy	Clinical features
General	Fixed lump Lash loss Change in size, shape and character Bleeding Ulceration
Basal cell carcinoma	Occurs in lower eyelid (50%), medial canthus (30%), upper eyelid (15%) and lateral canthus (5%) Nodular type: rolled, pearly edges, central umbilication and surrounded by dilated vessels Noduloulcerative: similar to nodular but with central ulceration Morphoea form: mildly elevated, flattish lesions with ill-defined borders
Squamous cell carcinoma	May mimic other lesions with flat, rolled edge, ulcerated or keratinised lesions
Malignant melanoma	Often pigmented and nodular, but occasional amelanotic and flat-spreading lentigo maligna type
Sebaceous cell carcinoma	Usually found on the upper lid Mimics many benign conditions, e.g. blepharitis and chalazion Occasionally, has a yellow discoloration May be multiple lesions
Merkel cell tumour (primary neuroendocrine carcinoma)	Solitary vascularised painless lump on upper eyelid

Table 6.8 Clinical features of eyelid malignancies

Investigations

Histopathology is essential in all lesions.

Differential diagnosis

Malignant lesions are often mistaken for each other, most commonly BCC and SCC, which can often only be distinguished

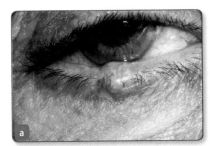

Figure 6.8 (a) Basal cell carcinoma. (b) Squamous cell carcinoma.

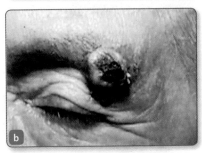

by histopathology. The presence of scaling correlates with hyperkeratosis and is associated with SCCs. Crusting occurs secondary to ulceration and exudation and is more strongly associated with BCCs. More dangerously, they are mistaken for benign lesions such as a chalazion, seborrhoeic keratosis and squamous papilloma. If there is any doubt, these cases should either be biopsied or followed closely for signs of malignancy.

Management

The vast majority of these tumours are treated surgically. The lowest recurrence rates are following **Mohs surgery**, in which all tumour margins in the excision specimen are examined and further specimens are taken until the defect is tumour free in order to preserve lid anatomy.

Conventional excision is adequate for small, primary, low-risk (particularly BCCs) skin tumours that are well circumscribed. If the wound cannot be closed directly, i.e. the defect requires a flap or graft, repair should be delayed until histological confirmation of the completeness of the tumour excision is obtained. For smaller BCCs, cryotherapy or localised chemotherapy with immune upregulators such as imiquimod can be used.

Radiotherapy and generalised chemotherapy is generally reserved for later metastatic disease, especially that involving the nerves, lymph nodes and orbit, and is often accompanied by surgical removal of orbital contents (**exenteration**) with lymph node dissection.

Prognosis

Prognosis varies with tumour type and the length of presentation. The peak time for recurrence is around 18 months postoperatively. Generally, BCC has a good outcome as it spreads by direct invasion and is generally a slow-growing tumour. The other malignant tumours are more aggressive and have higher 5-year mortality rates: SCC and malignant melanoma, 15% 5-year mortality; sebaceous cell carcinoma, 30% 5-year mortality.

6.8 Acquired nasolacrimal duct obstruction

Normally, tears travel down through the upper and lower puncta into the canaliculi, which join to form the common canaliculus. The common canaliculus empties into the lacrimal sac; the blink mechanism helps to pump tears into the nasolacrimal duct, which conducts the tears to the **inferior nasal meatus** – the opening of the nasolacrimal duct in the nose (see **Figure 6.1**). Blockage can occur anywhere along this pathway.

Epidemiology

Acquired nasolacrimal duct obstruction (ANLDO) is relatively common. Frequency increases with age, and it most commonly affects middle-aged to elderly women.

Causes

ANLDO has been classified into primary or secondary. Primary ANLDO is an idiopathic inflammatory process. Causes of secondary ANLDO are summarised in **Table 6.9**.

Pathogenesis

The exact cause of primary ANLDO has not been ascertained, but it is far more common in middle-aged and elderly women because of a narrower nasolacrimal duct. Postmenstrual changes have been proposed.

Secondary ANLDO can be caused by anything that blocks the lumen of the nasolacrimal duct, either internally, from its walls, or externally, by compression. The most common bacterial causes include *Actinomyces*, *Propionibacterium*, *Fusobacterium*, *Bacteroides*, *Mycobacterium* and *Chlamydia* species. Occasionally, infections may even cause stone formation. Common sites are the natural narrowings near the valves at either end of the nasolacrimal duct.

Infection of the lacrimal sac is termed acute dacrocystitis, which presents with a painful inflammatory swelling at the medial canthus that may be complicated by cellulitis or fistula formation.

Clinical features

It is important to examine the lids – position, blink, puncta and lashes – to exclude a secondary cause for the patient's epiphora

Causes	Type
Infection	Bacterial, viral, fungal
Inflammation	—
Trauma	—
Tumour	Primary or metastatic external tumour causing compression or primary nasolacrimal tumour

Table 6.9 Causes of secondary acquired nasolacrimal duct obstruction

(**Figure 3.4**). Pressure should be applied over the lacrimal sac area; if mucus or pus is seen regurgitating from the puncti, a mucocele is present. The skin over the sac area should be examined, specifically looking for a fistula.

Investigations

Diagnosis of the level of the obstruction of the lacrimal outflow tract is confirmed by a diagnostic lacrimal SWO (**Figure 6.9**). In this procedure, a blunt cannula is inserted through the lower punctum and fluid is gently irrigated; patients should be asked whether they feel the fluid in their nose or throat. If no fluid is felt, the cannula is carefully advanced until it is forced to stop. If there is a 'hard' stop (lacrimal bone, i.e. the cannula is in the sac) the obstruction is in the nasolacrimal duct. A 'soft' stop signifies the presence of a canalicular obstruction.

Differential diagnosis

For the differential diagnoses, see **Figure 3.4**.

Management

ANLDO should be treated conservatively if the patient's symptoms are mild or if the patient is infirm. Bouts of conjunctivitis can be treated with short courses of topical antibiotics; **dacrocystitis**, i.e. infection of the lacrimal sac, should be treated with oral antibiotics. When patients complain that symptoms are affecting their lifestyle or they have repeated infection, surgery can be considered.

The operations can be performed by either an ophthalmologist or an ENT surgeon. The basic principle of surgery is to

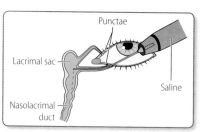

Figure 6.9 Nasolacrimal duct wash-out.

Punctae

Lacrimal sac

Saline

Nasolacrimal duct

fashion a new passage for tear outflow between the nasal cavity and the lacrimal sac, bypassing the obstruction (i.e. a dacrocytorhinostomy). This can be performed either externally via a skin incision or endoscopically in the nasal meatus. Often, following the procedure, a Silastic tube is placed in the lacrimal sac for several months to reduce the risk of the fistula closing.

Prognosis

Success following the operation varies from 80% to 95% by either skin incision or dacryocystorhinostomy.

Conjunctiva

Patients regularly present to both primary and secondary care with conjunctival diseases. The most common cause is infective conjunctivitis, which can become epidemic. These conditions are not usually sight threatening and, in most cases, result in minor annoyances. However, loss of the natural white colour of the eye often results in others noticing the conditions rather than patients themselves. The red eye is also a common response to other pathologies, and these have to be carefully screened for as differential diagnoses of conjunctival disease.

Anatomy and physiology

The conjunctiva is a mucous membrane that lines the sclera and the inner surface of the eyelids. Except at the tarsal plate, it is loosely attached to the underlying layers, which allows unrestricted movements of the globe. Goblet cells produce mucus, which, together with the aqueous secretions from the lacrimal gland and the oily secretions from the meibomian glands (tarsal glands), help lubricate the cornea and maintain its clarity.

7.1 Clinical scenario

Bilateral red eyes

Presentation

A 23-year-old woman presents to her GP's surgery with a 3-day history of bilateral red eyes (**Figure 7.1**).

Diagnostic approach

The red eye is a common cause of review for both GPs and ophthalmologists. This is a broad description covering several diseases. A good way to work through this is to think of causes from the front to the back of the eye. Asking more directed questions towards each of these anatomical locations in the history will quickly help to reduce the differential diagnoses.

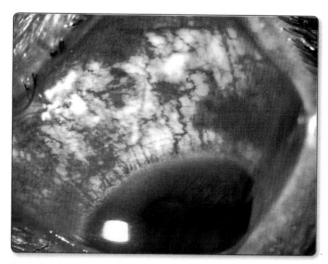

Figure 7.1 Patient's eye.

The patient describes bilateral red eye. Thus, many of the diagnoses are unlikely that are usually unilateral causes of redness, such as corneal foreign body. Among the possibilities are blepharitis, conjunctivitis and uveitis. Direct questioning about associated symptoms will help to narrow the diagnosis further (**Table 7.1**).

Further history

The patient states that she has been unwell with a sore throat for the past week. This follows an episode of her daughter also being unwell. The red eyes have gradually worsened over the last 3 days and are accompanied by a watery discharge. The patient's eyes are also burning; however, vision is not affected.

Diagnostic approach

Viral conjunctivitis is the most likely cause, especially with the prodromal symptoms. The aim is to examine for possible confirmatory signs, including preauricular lymph nodes and follicles under the eyelid. The other conditions, especially

Anatomical source	Disease	Symptoms
Lids	Blepharitis	Itchy, painful and crusty lids with gritty sensation
Conjunctiva	Subconjunctival haemorrhage	Onset usually without patient's knowledge. Asymptomatic
	Conjunctivitis	Viral type is usually bilateral, irritable and with watery discharge
Episclera	Episcleritis	Sudden-onset diffuse or focal redness that is mildly tender to touch and is usually accompanied by a foreign body sensation
Sclera	Scleritis	Can be diffuse or more commonly a localised area of extreme tenderness, described as a boring pain that often keeps patients awake at night
Cornea	Keratitis	Vision may be reduced, and there is a foreign body sensation, photophobia and tearing
Uvea	Uveitis	Photophobia and vision is reduced; can be bilateral

Table 7.1 Common causes of red eye with associated symptoms

blepharitis, can easily be excluded by ophthalmic examination of the lids.

Examination
The patient's temperature is 39°C and she has preauricular lymphadenopathy.

Ophthalmic examination: For a summary of the ophthalmic examination, see **Table 7.2**.

Diagnostic approach
The normal vision and follicles under the lid with a normal lid margin exclude severe blepharitis and confirm viral conjunctivitis. Further confirmation can be made by taking a viral swab from the conjunctiva.

	Right eye		Left eye
6/6	**Visual acuity**	6/6	
No response to direct and consensual reflex	**Pupil**	Normal direct and consensual reflex	
Lid margins clear	**Lid**	Lid margins clear	
Clear	**Cornea**	Clear	
Injected throughout Watery discharge Follicles under lid	**Conjunctiva**	Injected throughout Watery discharge Follicles under lid	
Clear	**Anterior chamber**	Clear	
Clear	**Lens**	Clear	
Clear	**Vitreous**	Clear	
Clear view of fundus	**Fundus**	Clear view of fundus	

Table 7.2 Ophthalmic examination: results for a patient who presented with bilateral red eyes

7.2 Infective conjunctivitis

Conjunctivitis is inflammation of the conjunctiva. Infective conjunctivitis is one of the most common causes for bilateral red eye.

Epidemiology

Infective conjunctivitis is a very common condition, resulting in one third of eye cases seen by GPs. It is more common among children, who can rapidly spread infection at school or nursery. There is also a peak in occurrence among the elderly.

Causes

For the causes of conjunctivitis, see **Table 7.3**.

Type of infective conjunctivitis	Common pathogens	Signs and symptoms
Bacterial (**Figure 7.2**)	Gram-positive cocci: *Staphylococcus Streptococcus* spp. Gram-negative cocci: *Neisseria meningitidis Neisseria gonorrhoeae* Gram-negative rods: *Haemophilus* spp. *Chlamydia trachomatis*	Acute red eye Thick mucopurulent discharge
Viral (**Figure 7.3**)	Adenovirus Herpes simplex Enterovirus Coxsackievirus	Itchy Watery discharge Associated recent intercurrent viral illness Follicles seen under the lid with preauricular lymphadenopathy common Rarely, corneal opacities Usually resolves in 2 weeks
Chlamydial (**Figure 7.4**)	*Chlamydia trachomatis*	Mild injection Moderate thickish discharge Recent unprotected sexual activity Preauricular lymphadenopathy Follicles under lid Symptoms >2 weeks Slow onset Poor response to antibiotics ± genital discharge

Table 7.3 Differentiating causative organisms; signs and symptoms of types of conjunctivitis

Pathogenesis

As with other tissue affected by infective pathogens, the body mounts an immune response, resulting in inflammation. This leads to the hyperaemia and discharge commonly seen in conjunctivitis.

Clinical features

For most patients, conjunctivitis is usually a transitory irritation; however, a focused history is required to rule out more damaging causes of conjunctivitis, including gonococcal and chlamydial (**Figure 7.4**) causes. The diagnosis can generally be made without the need for specialist equipment. Almost all patients complain of others noticing a red eye (**Figure 7.3**). Other patients will complain of discharge (**Figure 7.2**) and occasional grittiness. Certain broad differences occur between the various causes (**Table 7.2**).

Investigations

If conjunctivitis persists for longer than 7–10 days, a swab should be taken to check for viral and bacterial causes and chlamydia.

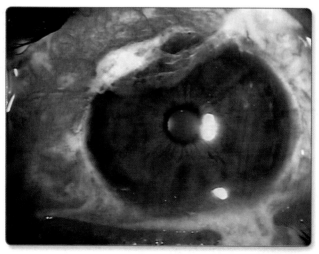

Figure 7.2 Purulent discharge in bacterial conjunctivitis.

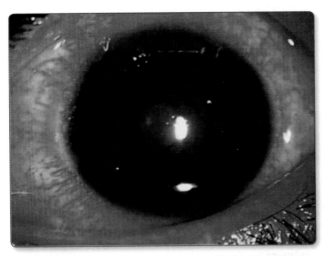

Figure 7.3 Red eye in viral conjunctivitis with some subepithelial corneal opacities.

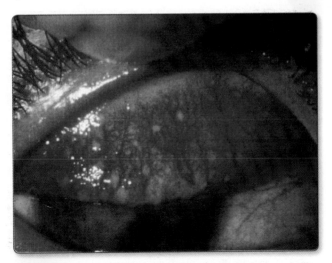

Figure 7.4 Follicles under the lid in chlamydial conjunctivitis.

Differential diagnosis

Differential diagnoses include other causes of acute red eye (see **Figure 3.1**).

Management

Infective conjunctivitis should be managed conservatively for the first 5–7 days as it generally resolves by itself. Patients generally need to be counselled that symptoms resolve in the majority of cases and that treatment will make little or no difference. Viral causes make up approximately two thirds of cases of infective conjunctivitis.

Patients should be advised to wash their hands after touching their eyes and to use separate towels from others in the household to prevent spread. Children with conjunctivitis are generally excluded from school or nursery until discharge stops.

Severe symptoms

If symptoms are severe, an antibiotic may be prescribed as this can speed recovery in bacterial conjunctivitis by a day on average. However, if there are danger signs such as hyperacute purulent conjunctivitis or chronic conjunctivitis with a history of recent unprotected intercourse with a new partner, swabs should be taken and treatment instigated sooner. Initially, this will be with a broad-spectrum topical antibiotic, such as fucithalmic or chloramphenicol. Photophobia is a sure sign of corneal involvement, and, in these cases, a weak topical corticosteroid such as betamethasone can be used four times a day.

Chlamydia and gonorrhoea

Chlamydial conjunctivitis is a sexually transmitted disease in developed countries and can result in spread and secondary infertility among women; consequently, both male and female partners should be treated and referred to the genitourinary clinic.

Gonococcal conjunctivitis causes severe hyperacute hyperpurulent conjunctivitis that can result in a rapid keratitis; it is also highly infectious and requires case tracing and treatment follow-up. Both these conditions require systemic treatment.

Prognosis

The prognosis is generally very good for most types of conjunctivitis, with two thirds of cases resolving within 5 days with or without treatment.

7.3 Allergic conjunctivitis

Allergic conjunctivitis is an inflammation of the conjunctiva instigated by an allergen. Allergic conjunctivitis is divided chronologically and more loosely by type. **Perennial conjunctivitis** occurs throughout the year whereas seasonal allergic conjunctivitis occurs in defined seasons. **Vernal conjunctivitis** is a chronic bilateral conjunctivitis affecting the young with marked seasonal variation whereas **atopic conjunctivitis** is linked to a history of atopic disease with less seasonal variation.

Epidemiology

Allergic conjunctivitis is a common condition in its various forms. Up to one fifth of the population is thought to have had allergic conjunctivitis at some point. There is little variation among perennial and seasonal types, but the vernal and atopic allergic types of conjunctivitis are more commonly found among boys and teenagers.

Causes

Specific allergens are most associated with perennial and seasonal allergic conjunctivitis. These include various air-borne particles. Pollen is a common cause of seasonal allergic conjunctivitis. The type of pollen varies with season, with tree pollen being most common in late spring to early summer, grass pollen in mid- to late summer and ragweed common later in summer. Perennial allergic conjunctivitis can be triggered by a variety of persistent allergens, including pollution, pet dander and dust mites.

Both vernal and atopic conjunctivitis are closely linked to atopic disease.

Pathogenesis

The primary immune cell involved is the mast cell. On encountering an allergen, these cells degranulate, releasing a number of mediators including histamines, proteases and cyclo-oxygenase. The direct and downstream effects on these lead to nerve activation and itching, blood vessel dilation and increased blood vessel permeability. Later, a chronic inflammatory reaction ensues, with persistent activation involving lymphocytic proliferation.

Clinical features

The types of allergic conjunctivitis are often difficult to differentiate, but a detailed history of timings of irritation, an understanding of the epidemiology of the diseases and examination clues may help.

Patients with all types of allergic conjunctivitis have varying degrees of itchiness, eye watering and redness. Examination classically reveals hyperaemia, lid oedema and conjunctival swelling.

Vernal conjunctivitis is most active in spring and has a whitish discharge. Examination sometimes reveals white spots known as Tranta dots at the limbus and large papillae under the eyelids (**Figure 7.5**). If severe, direct contact of the cornea with the inflamed tarsal conjunctiva may lead to corneal ulceration.

In atopic conjunctivitis, the face and periocular skin may have an eczematous rash. The lid margins show blepharitis and are often encrusted with bacteria. Papillae are common and predominate inferiorly with occasional vascularisation of the cornea.

Investigations

Investigations are rarely required to confirm the diagnosis except in severe and persistent cases in which the diagnosis is in doubt.

Differential diagnosis

Differential diagnoses include other causes of conjunctivitis and dry eye. The most difficult to differentiate are viral and

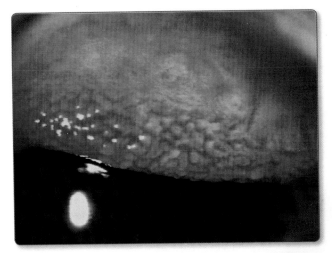

Figure 7.5 Papillae seen under the eyelids of a patient with vernal allergic conjunctivitis.

chlamydial causes. Both these conditions can result in some itching and lid swelling. However, these causes generally lead to follicle formation and also tender preauricular lymphadenopathy.

Management

The treatment of the various types of allergic conjunctivitis is similar, with considerations made for severity and the age of patients.

In mild cases, no treatment is required. Perennial types and seasonal types can initially be treated as in hayfever with systemic antihistamines. However, children with vernal types have to be watched closely for quick progression. Atopic and vernal types and more severe perennial/seasonal conjunctivitis are treated with topical mast cell stabilisers and topical non-steroidal medication. However, usually by the time of presentation, a mast cell-independent inflammation has been incited and a short course of corticosteroid drops is required to dampen down the inflammation.

Mast cell stabilisers such as sodium cromoglycate and nedocromil sodium are then used for prevention to reduce recurrence, with weak corticosteroids such as betamethasone and fluorometholone used for control of flare-ups when they occur.

In the most severe cases, direct subconjunctival corticosteroids injection is used.

Prognosis

Patients should be counselled to use preventative treatment prior to expected periods of exacerbation. Atopic and vernal keratoconjunctivitis are more likely to result in complications, such as early cataract and **keratoconus** and ectasia of the cornea resulting from chronic rubbing.

7.4 Subconjunctival haemorrhage

The conjunctiva is a transparent mucous membrane lining the lids and globe. It is traversed by vessels that lie under its surface. **Subconjunctival haemorrhage** results when these vessels bleed into the layer under the conjunctiva and above the white sclera.

Epidemiology

Subconjunctival haemorrhage is a common condition. Its occurrence increases with age.

Causes

The causes of subconjunctival haemorrhage can be:
- idiopathic
- traumatic, e.g. direct trauma, secondary to surgery or rubbing
- hypertension, e.g. systemic or localised due to the Valsalva manoeuvre
- bleeding disorders, e.g. hepatic disease, vitamin C deficiency

Pathogenesis

Bleeding results from breakage of conjunctival and episcleral vessels. This is due to direct insult, increased intraluminal pressure, inherent deficiencies in the wall of the vessels or defects in blood vessel repair processes.

Clinical features

Patients often complain of a red eye. Most commonly, this is something that others have commented on and the patients are asymptomatic or have a dull ache. Examination usually reveals a pink or red patch of blood under the conjunctiva, occasionally resulting in lifting of the conjunctiva (**Figure 7.6**). Unless caused by trauma, this is usually non-tender to gentle palpation. A history of trauma warrants a complete examination of the eye. Patients should also be asked about other bleeding episodes elsewhere in the body to assess the risk for bleeding disorders.

Investigations

No investigations are normally required. In rare cases of recurrent subconjunctival haemorrhage of unknown cause, further blood pressure measurements, full blood count, liver function tests and coagulation profile can be taken to screen for bleeding disorders.

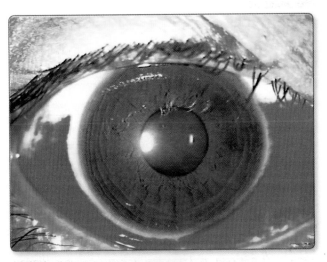

Figure 7.6 Subconjunctival haemorrhage.

Differential diagnosis

The differential diagnoses include other causes of red eye:

- *conjunctivitis*: usually covering the whole conjunctiva; there is also discharge
- *anterior uveitis*: patients have photophobia and a miosed pupil and the eye is tender to palpation
- *episcleritis*: patients report discomfort when the eye is touched; the red eye can be blanched with administration of 10% phenylephrine drops
- *scleritis*: patients report severe pain and the eye is extremely tender to touch

Management

Patients should be reassured, usually with an explanation that this is similar to a bruise on the eye. Unnecessary use of aspirin or non-steroidal anti-inflammatory drugs should be avoided. As the vessels are more friable, eye rubbing should also be avoided. The haemorrhage usually resolves in 7–10 days.

Prognosis

The prognosis is very good with no lasting sequelae.

Cornea and sclera

Corneal disease, especially dry eye, is a common phenomenon. The incidence of infectious disease is also increasing with the use of contact lenses. Generally, these conditions have similar symptomatology, which is linked to the activation of fine corneal nerves and their default response. Symptoms include foreign body sensation/grittiness, photophobia and tearing. These conditions are irritating in their mild forms, but can potentially be sight threatening by causing opacity of the normally clear cornea.

Scleral and episcleral diseases are inflammatory in nature. They are important because they are often difficult to differentiate from each other. Scleritis – the severe form – can result in loss of both vision and the eye.

Anatomy and histology

The outer layer of the globe is composed of collagenous fibres that constitute the sclera posteriorly and the cornea anteriorly. The particular orientation of the collagen fibres in the cornea confers clarity, which is maintained by the continual resurfacing of the corneal epithelium by tears.

The cornea is composed of three layers from superficial to deep: epithelium, stroma and endothelium. Each layer is separated from the next by a membrane – the anterior limiting lamina (Bowman's membrane) anteriorly and the posterior limiting lamina (Descemet's membrane) posteriorly. An aperture in the sclera posteriorly allows the retinal ganglion cell axons to leave the eye as the optic nerve. The anterior one third of the sclera is lined by conjunctiva externally whilst the posterior two thirds is lined by the choroid and ciliary body internally. Blood supply is from deep and superficial episcleral vessels externally and the choroid internally.

8.1 Clinical scenario

Sharp pain in the eye

Presentation

A 25-year-old woman presents to her GP with a 2-day history of sharp pain in the right eye.

Diagnostic approach

Symptoms which have an ocular cause are inevitably accompanied by detectable abnormalities on clinical examination. The sharp character of the pain indicates a problem with the surface of the eye, especially the cornea. Scleritis presents with pain that is typically described as being dull. It is useful to try to define the characteristics of any ocular pain as this often has diagnostic value, enabling the clinician to localise the lesion anatomically (**Table 8.1**).

Further history

The patient has had no specific discharge, but her eye is tearing and she has a foreign body sensation. Bright lights also make the pain worse. The eye has become increasingly red over the last day.

Previous ocular history: The patient wears monthly disposable contact lenses for myopia.

Diagnostic approach

Photophobia is a diagnostically useful symptom (or sign) and is associated with keratitis or iritis (see **Figure 3.1**). In this clinical

Anatomical location	Pain characteristics
Conjunctiva	Burning and watering
Cornea	Sharp knife-like pain with associated foreign body sensation, photophobia and tearing
Sclera	Boring pain at the back of the eye; severe tenderness to touch
Anterior uvea	Ache with photophobia and visual blurring

Table 8.1 Common characteristics of pain with anatomical location

setting, the most likely cause is keratitis, which is strongly associated with the use of contact lenses.

Often, patients who are photophobic are extremely difficult to examine; in these cases, instillation of a topical anaesthetic such as oxybuprocaine can be diagnostically and therapeutically useful. If the pain and photophobia resolve, the symptoms must have arisen from the cornea and conjunctiva as only these structures have been anaesthetised. It is mandatory to instil fluorescein into any eye(s) that are red or painful to detect abnormalities in the corneal epithelium.

The examination can be performed with a +10 lens on a handheld ophthalmoscope to magnify any corneal changes.

Examination

For further information on the examination, see **Figure 8.1**.

Ophthalmic examination: The ophthalmic examination includes a localised inferior injection. For a summary of the remaining ophthalmic examination, see **Table 8.2**.

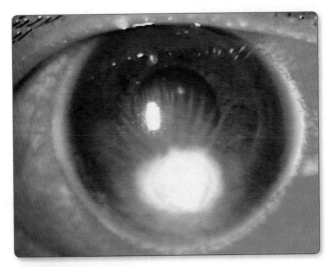

Figure 8.1 Corneal infiltrate and ulcer.

	Right eye		Left eye
	6/12	**Visual acuity**	6/6
	Normal direct and consensual reflex	**Pupil**	Normal direct and consensual reflex
	Infiltrate inferiorly near the centre Fluorescein highlights ulcer over infiltrate (**Figure 8.1**)	**Cornea**	Clear
	Quiet	**Anterior chamber**	Quiet

Table 8.2 Ophthalmic examination: results for a patient who presented with sharp pain in the eye

Diagnostic approach

The patient's presentation is most likely to be caused by a bacterial keratitis secondary to contact lens wear. Contact lens wear can confer an increased risk of severity, with different bacteria involved. Investigations and definitive diagnosis can be made by corneal scrape and culture (see section 8.3).

8.2 Dry eye

Dry eye is a multifactorial disease. The tear film (**Figure 1.15**) is composed of three layers, each produced by secretions from the conjunctiva, lids and lacrimal gland. The outer layer is a lipid-rich layer produced mainly by secretions from the meibomian glands (tarsal glands). This layer reduces tear evaporation. The middle layer is an aqueous layer, which provides the main bulk of tear film volume and is produced by the lacrimal gland and the accessory lacrimal glands (gland of Wolfring and gland of Krause). Finally, a mucin-rich base layer produced by the conjunctival goblet cells enables tears to attach and spread over the conjunctival surface.

The tear film can be disrupted by deficiencies or defects in any or all of these layers, resulting in the symptoms of dry eye.

Epidemiology

Tear film abnormalities are a major cause of patients attending both primary care and specialist eye care. Of this population, 10–30% are affected by symptoms of dry eye.

Causes

The causes of dry eye include the following (adapted from the Dry Eye Workshop 2007 classification):

1. Sjögren syndrome – aqueous reduction
   - primary
   - secondary
2. Non-Sjögren syndrome dry eye
   - primary lacrimal gland deficiencies
   - secondary lacrimal gland deficiencies
   - obstruction of the lacrimal gland ducts
   - reflex hyposecretion
3. Evaporative dry eye with tear dysfunction
   - intrinsic causes: meibomian gland dysfunction; low blink rate, e.g. secondary to facial nerve palsy
   - extrinsic causes: ocular surface disorders; contact lens wear; ocular surface disease

Pathogenesis

The pathogenesis varies as to the cause. The most common cause of dry eye, meibomian gland dysfunction, is thought to be caused by hormonal changes occurring at menopause.

Sjögren syndrome is an autoimmune disease of the lacrimal and salivary glands resulting from destruction secondary to lymphocytic infiltration. Other causes, including neurogenic loss and contact lens wear, reduce reflex tear production by reduced corneal sensation.

Clinical features

Patients complain of dryness of the eyes and, depending on the severity, pain, redness, photophobia and foreign body sensation. Generally, in true dryness, there is no tear overspill. However, in tear film dysfunction, wind or cold may induce increased reflex tearing as the tear film does not protect the cornea owing to evaporation paradoxically inducing more tearing.

The history should include a review of associated conditions, including:

- rheumatoid arthritis
- connective tissue disorders
- diabetes
- Sjögren syndrome

The majority of the examination can be performed using fluorescein dye without specialist equipment. Signs of dry eye include reduced tear film height, early break-up (<10 s), corneal epithelial defects, conjunctival injection at the limbus and mucin plaques or strings. Corneal sensation should be tested for neurogenic loss.

Investigations

The Schirmer test is used as an approximate measure of dryness. This is performed by placing a strip of filter paper in the inferior fornix and asking the patient to close their eyes for 5 min. Normal is >10 mm of wetting; moderate dryness is 5–10 mm; and severe deficiency is <5 mm.

A blood sample should be taken and tested for antinuclear, anti-Ro, anti-La and antineutrophil cytoplasm antibodies and rheumatoid factor.

Differential diagnosis

Other causes of symptoms include a foreign body or trichiasis, which can be ruled out by examination.

Management

Treatment recommendations are usually undertaken in a stepwise fashion according to dry eye severity (**Table 8.3**).

Dry eye severity	Management
Mild/episodic; occurs under environmental stress	Education, environmental, dietary modifications Elimination of offending systemic medications Artificial tears at night Eyelid steam massage if meibomian gland plugging
Moderate episodic or chronic; stress or no stress	Artificial tears at night Oral tetracyclines (for meibomianitis and rosacea) Temporary punctal plugs
Severe frequent/constant pain without stress	Bandage protection contact lenses Permanent punctal occlusion with cautery
Severe/disabling and constant	Systemic anti-inflammatory agents Surgery including: Tarsorrhaphy Mucous membrane grafting Amniotic membrane transplantation

Table 8.3 Treatment strategy for dry eyes based on severity. Adapted from the Dry Eye Workshop 2007 classification (Ocular Surface 2007;5:163–78)

Referral to a rheumatologist is warranted to rule out other connective tissue disorders or in cases of confirmed Sjögren syndrome.

Prognosis
Generally, the prognosis is good once suitable tear substitutes are identified. Patients need to be counselled to continue using treatments in the absence of symptoms as a preventative measure.

8.3 Infectious keratitis
Infectious keratitis is a serious, potentially blinding, condition resulting from bacterial, viral, fungal and protozoal infection to the cornea.

Epidemiology

Incidence rates have been reported at between 6 and 700 per 100,000 per year. When cultured, approximately 50% of ulcers will provide positive results. Bacterial keratitis was found to be more common among young contact lens wearers. However, the elderly were more likely to have severe blinding disease owing to late presentation and poor immune response. Fungal keratitis is more common among adults and in warmer tropical climates.

Causes

For a list of causes of infectious keratitis, see **Table 8.4**.

Pathogenesis

The chief mechanism of entry for bacteria, fungi and protozoa is via a defect in the corneal epithelium. In the stroma, the

Type	Most common causes
Bacterial	Gram positive: Coagulase-negative *Staphylococcus* *Streptococcus pneumoniae* *Staphylococcus aureus* Gram negative: *Pseudomonas aeruginosa* Enterobacteriaceae *Moraxella* *Haemophilus* *Neisseria gonorrhoeae*
Viral	Herpes simplex type 1 Herpes zoster Adenovirus
Fungal	Filamentous: *Fusarium* *Aspergillus* Yeasts: *Candida* spp. *Cryptococcus* spp.
Protozoa	Acanthamoeba

Table 8.4 Causes of infectious keratitis

infecting organisms proliferate and induce necrosis, leading to ulceration and thinning of the cornea. Neutrophil recruitment leads to further necrosis before cytokine release leads to further inflammatory cell recruitment, which leads to infiltrates on the cornea and hypopyon.

Herpetic keratitis results from a primary skin or mucous membrane infection due to the virus travelling to the trigeminal nerve. Reactivation in the cornea leads to the virus travelling via the ophthalmic division of the trigeminal nerve to the corneal nerve.

Clinical features

Patients have severe pain, photophobia, foreign body sensation and loss of vision. The history should include a careful assessment of the risk factors, including contact lens wear, trauma, dry eyes and blepharitis, and a systemic history, e.g. immunosuppression caused by diabetes mellitus.

Patients who are unable to open their eyes are often easiest to examine with a small amount of local anaesthetic. Examination using fluorescein dye will reveal a red eye with an ulcer. Often, a white corneal infiltrate is seen. In severe cases, a hypopyon can be seen as a white fluid level (**Figure 8.2**).

Generally, there are very few distinguishing features on clinical examination between type, and diagnosis is made by culture. However, patients with acanthamoeba keratitis develop a mid-peripheral ring infiltrate and have severe pain, and those with fungal keratitis can develop multiple satellite lesions. Herpetic keratitis classically presents with a dendritic pattern (**Figure 8.3**).

Risks

The risks include:

- extended wear contact lenses
- ocular surface disease, such as dry eye
- blepharitis
- diabetes mellitus
- rheumatoid arthritis
- loss of the corneal reflex
- use of topical corticosteroids or traditional healing medications

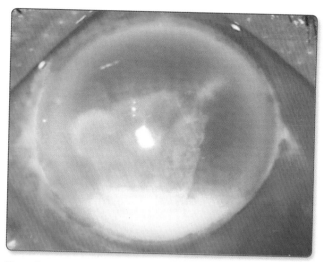

Figure 8.2 Severe bacterial keratitis.

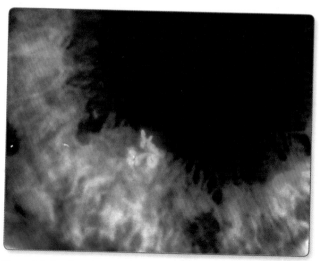

Figure 8.3 Dendritic ulcer in herpes simplex keratitis.

Investigations

Samples should be taken under topical anaesthesia with a sterile needle from the edge of the ulcer and placed on a microscope slide; they should be assessed immediately by Gram staining and microscopy, and plated in blood and chocolate agar for bacteria and Sabouraud medium for fungal growth.

Suspicion of acanthamoeba requires growth of samples on agar plates seeded with *Escherichia coli*.

Differential diagnosis

Differential diagnoses include other causes for corneal ulceration, such as marginal keratitis (usually only in the peripheral cornea and with associated blepharitis) and corneal abrasion (history of sudden pain or trauma leaving purely a discrete epithelial defect) as well as the other differential diagnoses for red eye (see **Figure 3.1**).

Management

Early empirical treatment with close follow-up is key. Specific treatment can be instituted as results are received. Initial therapy is with a broad-spectrum quinolone, e.g. exocin, or dual therapy with a cephalosporin, e.g. cefuroxime, and aminoglycoside, e.g. gentamicin, to cover the most common pathogens.

Fungal keratitis is treated with topical and oral antifungal drugs, such as amphotericin or ketoconazole.

Acanthamoeba requires several months of treatment with propamidine or hexamidine in combination with polyhexamethylene biguanide or chlorhexidine.

Herpes simplex epithelial keratitis disease is treated with topical aciclovir ointment. In herpetic stromal keratitis, topical corticosteroids are used to reduce inflammation with topical or oral aciclovir cover.

If the cornea is severely scarred, corneal transplant may be indicated once infection is cleared to restore vision.

Prognosis

The prognosis is good for patients presenting early with mildly pathogenic species of bacteria and herpetic disease. However, the elderly, contact lens wearers and those with fungal keratitis have an increased risk of visual debilitation.

Patients with herpetic disease must be counselled about recurrence while contact lens wearers should be counselled about the length of daily wear, hygiene and type of contact lens being worn.

8.4 Scleritis/episcleritis

Scleritis is inflammation of the sclera. Scleritis is often divided anatomically into anterior and posterior types (**Table 8.5**).

Episcleritis is a more benign and superficial inflammation involving mainly the superficial episcleral vessels.

Epidemiology

Scleritis is a relatively uncommon disease, with a prevalence of approximately 6 per 100,000. It is twice as common among women as among men and occurs most commonly in the fifth to seventh decades.

Causes

The associations of scleritis are summarised in **Table 8.6**.

Pathogenesis

Scleritis is a T-cell-driven inflammation with recruitment of other inflammatory cells such macrophages. Necrotising granulomas have been identified, leading to scleral thinning.

Anatomical location	Type	Subtype
Anterior	Diffuse	–
	Nodular	–
	Necrotising	Inflammatory
		Non-inflammatory (scleromalacia perforans)
Posterior scleritis	–	–

Table 8.5 Classification of scleritis

Type of condition	Examples
Idiopathic	—
Inflammatory	Rheumatoid arthritis Wegener granulomatosis Ankylosing spondylitis Polyarteritis nodosa Sarcoidosis Systemic lupus erythematosus
Infectious	Syphilis Herpes simplex Varicella Bacterial, mycobacterial, fungal and amoebal infection
Other	Induced by surgery/trauma

Table 8.6 Conditions associated with scleritis

Clinical features

Patients typically present with a red eye and pain. The pain is described as varying from mild to a dull ache but more commonly as a boring pain that wakes patients at night. Examination reveals a red eye with focal redness and, more rarely, a diffuse redness throughout the eye. Patients are exquisitely tender on palpation of the dilated vessels. Posterior scleritis displays no anterior signs of activity. However, it may result in retinal changes, changes to the muscle insertions and orbital inflammation. These present as reduced vision with subretinal fluid, diplopia and proptosis.

Episcleritis is most commonly painless. Patients may complain of an ache and gritty sensation.

When associated with rheumatoid arthritis, scleritis may lead to thinning of the sclera and perforation.

Investigations

A blood sample should be taken to exclude associated conditions in scleritis. Tests include:
- a full blood count, antinuclear antibodies and rheumatoid factor measurement
- measurement of antineutrophil cytoplasmic antibodies

- a syphilitic screen
- Lyme disease serology

In addition, the erythrocyte sedimentation rate can be used for monitoring.

If posterior scleritis is suspected, an ultrasound scan may reveal fluid at the back of the eye under the Tenon capsule (fascial sheath of the eyeball). When this occurs around the optic nerve, it is called the 'T' sign.

Episcleritis does not need investigation.

> ## Clinical insight
>
> To differentiate scleritis from episcleritis, which is a much milder disease, phenylephrine 10% can be instilled in the eye. After several minutes, the deep dilated episcleral vessels will remain dilated in scleritis, whereas the superficial episcleral vessels will constrict, causing blanching, in episcleritis.

Differential diagnosis

Differential diagnoses include other causes of red eye (see **Figure 3.1**).

Management

A stepwise pattern of prescribing is often used. Episcleritis and diffuse and nodular anterior scleritis resolve with oral non-steroidal anti-inflammatory drugs (NSAIDs) alone in the majority of cases. Drugs include a 2-week course of flurbiprofen or indometacin. Treatment can be supplemented by topical NSAIDs and corticosteroids.. When NSAIDs are ineffective, a short course of a high-dose corticosteroids. is used, e.g. 0.5–1 mg of prednisolone per kilogram bodyweight for a week and tailoring the dose to the response.

For necrotising and posterior scleritis, treatment is with pulsed methylprednisolone (1 g) over 3 days before switching to oral prednisolone at a dose of 0.5–1 mg per kilogram bodyweight. Non-steroidal immunosuppressive therapy is instituted if treatment with corticosteroids. is likely to be prolonged, which is commonly the case with necrotising types.

Prognosis

The prognosis varies as to the type of scleritis. Diffuse and nodular anterior types are unlikely to cause visual disturbance.

Those patients with posterior scleritis and necrotising anterior scleritis are most likely to have visual disturbance culminating in perforation with scleromalacia perforans.

Episcleritis usually resolves with no sequelae.

Diseases of the lens

Lens disease represents one of the most common causes of treatable blindness in the world. The majority of these cases are in the developing world, where rapidly increasing populations and inadequate health infrastructure mean that many people remain untreated. Concerted efforts have been made to tackle the increasing problem through programmes such as the World Health Organization's Vision 2020 programme.

Anatomy and physiology

The normal lens consists of an outer elastic capsule, soft cortex and a dense central nucleus (**Figure 1.11**). The lens is normally clear owing to the formation of crystalline lens fibres that are laid down over time by lens epithelial cells. These fibres are aligned in such a way as to allow light to pass through. The fibres are not replaced but added to, and the inner fibres continue to be compressed.

The lens is attached to the ciliary body via collagenous fibres in the zonules that attach to the capsule. These fibres allow the muscles of the ciliary body to alter the shape of the lens to help focus light rays onto the retina.

9.1 Clinical scenario

Gradually reducing vision

Presentation

A 70-year-old man presents to the ophthalmic outpatient department with gradually reducing vision in the right eye.

Diagnostic approach

Reduced vision can potentially be caused by any element of the ocular system and visual pathway. A structured approach following the pathway of light from the outside of the eye to the retina and then on to the visual pathway may help diagnosis. It is important to remember that the most common cause for the symptoms is a change of refraction. This can be excluded by pinhole testing during examination.

Diagnostic clues in the history The bilateral and gradual reduction in vision immediately rules out conditions that are likely to affect one eye at a time, such as retinal detachment, and those that are more acute, such as temporal arteritis or retinal detachment.

Further history

The patient's vision is globally reduced in the right eye and has worsened over months. This has affected his driving for distance vision and reading for near vision. He also has problems with glare, but has not noticed any new floaters or flashing lights.

Previous ocular history: The patient has been using reading glasses for reading.

Diagnostic approach

A handheld fundoscope set at +10 can be used to exclude corneal abnormalities. In addition, this can also be used to examine for cataract after dilating with tropicamide 1%. If the vitreous is involved then the retina may not be seen despite a clear lens. Finally, dilated fundoscopy can be used to examine the retina and optic nerve (see **Figure 3.2**).

Examination

The patient's eye is shown in **Figure 9.1**.

Ophthalmic examination: For a summary of the ophthalmic examination, see **Table 9.1**.

Diagnostic approach

The examination quite clearly shows a cataract to be the cause of loss of vision. All structures behind the cataract are difficult to visualise. Of note, the pinhole corrects for only one line. If the reduction in vision was due to refraction in a patient with previously normal vision, one would expect a three- or four-line improvement on the Snellen chart.

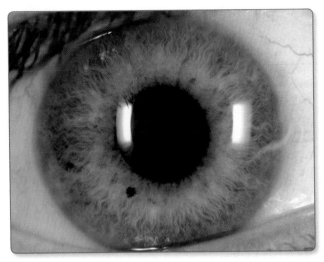

Figure 9.1 The eye of a patient with gradually reducing vision.

Right eye		Left eye
	Visual acuity	
6/24	**Distance unaided**	6/6
6/18	**Pinhole**	6/6
N18	**Near**	N6
Normal direct and consensual reflex	**Pupil**	Normal direct and consensual reflex
Clear	**Cornea**	Clear
Clear	**Anterior chamber**	Clear
Opacity on red reflex Whitening	**Lens**	Clear
Unable to see clearly	**Vitreous**	Clear
Poor view of fundus	**Fundus**	Clear view of fundus
Difficult view but appears normal	**Disc**	Normal vessels and disc

Table 9.1 Ophthalmic examination: results for a patient who presented with gradually reducing vision

9.2 Cataract

Cataract is an opacity in the crystalline lens.

Epidemiology

Cataracts are the most common cause of blindness in the world, with 90% of cases occurring in the developing world. It is estimated that the number of people affected worldwide by blindness caused by cataract will reach 75 million by 2020.

Causes

For the causes of cataract, see **Table 9.2**.

Pathogenesis

Laying down of fibres results in sclerosis of the nucleus. Pigment is also laid down, causing a gradual browning of the lens. A combination of factors, including ultraviolet light exposure, is thought to result in oxidative stress altering the protein structure of the lens and causing the lens to become opaque.

Clinical features

Patients with senile cataract usually have gradual loss of vision. This is most often noted when a normal activity of daily living

Type	Causes
Congenital	Infection: rubella, measles, herpes simplex, varicella, Epstein–Barr virus, syphilis, toxoplasma Genetic: familial, trisomy 21, galactosaemia
Acquired	Ageing Malnutrition Ultraviolet light exposure Toxicity, e.g. smoking Systemic disease, e.g. diabetes Drugs, e.g. corticosteroids Eye disease, e.g. myopia, glaucoma, uveitis Trauma

Table 9.2 Causes of cataract

such as reading or driving becomes progressively difficult. Patients may also complain of glare when looking at lights; this is caused by the scatter of light. Cataractous lenses also have increased refractive power causing increasing short sightedness – a phenomenon known as myopic shift.

Near and distant vision and contrast sensitivity are reduced. Examination usually reveals a whitening of the lens. This is noted when looking at the pupil. In all cases it is important to examine the whole eye to exclude other causes for a reduction in vision, e.g. macular degeneration. If the fundus cannot be seen, a test for relative afferent pupil defect can be carried out to rule out optic nerve abnormalities. A cataract alone cannot cause a relative afferent pupillary defect.

> ## Clinical insight
>
> Cataracts can be seen more clearly using a fundoscope set at +10.

Diagnostic criteria

The three main types of cataract are nuclear sclerotic (**Figure 9.2**), cortical (**Figure 9.3**) and posterior subcapsular (**Figure 9.4**).

Investigations

Investigations are not usually required for senile cataract. If there is no clear view of the fundus, an ultrasound is used to ensure that the retina is intact and that there is no malignant pathology.

When a decision to operate is made, an ultrasound, to measure eye length, and keratometry, to measure corneal curvature, are used to help calculate appropriate intraocular lens power.

Management

Cataract is not an ophthalmic emergency except in the very young, when amblyopia can result, and in rare instances when the cataractous lens results in high intraocular pressure or inflammation. It is irreversible; therefore, surgery is required to remove cataract. A decision about whether to operate depends on a multitude of factors. Primarily, this is a balance between patients' visual needs and the risks of surgery. Patients who

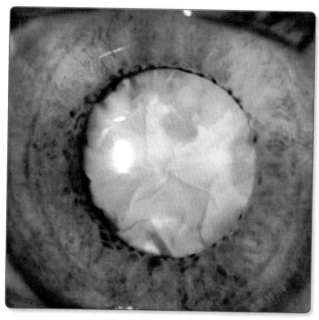

Figure 9.2 A nuclear sclerotic cataract.

have a reduction in vision and do not wish to undergo surgery often find low-vision aids useful.

Prognosis

The prognosis is generally very good as long as there is no coexisting pathology. Treatment results in 90% of patients achieving driving vision.

9.3 Cataract surgery

Cataract surgery has been practised in some form since the sixth century BC. It is the most commonly performed surgical procedure worldwide, with approximately 10 million operations performed each year. The aim is to remove the cataractous lens and to replace this with an artificial intraocular lens.

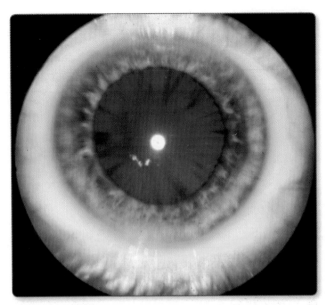

Figure 9.3 A cortical cataract.

The procedure and type of lens inserted varies according to available resources.

Investigations

In the developed world, a preoperative visit includes:

- examination of vision and a full eye examination
- examination of the eyelids for possible risk of infection
- examination of the cornea for clarity during the operation
- assessment of the density of the cataract and exclusion of other pathology to make a fair assessment of possible visual outcome
- obtaining consent
- **biometry**, i.e. ultrasound to measure the length of the eye
- **keratometry**, i.e. measurement of the corneal curvature; this aids the choice of the intraocular lens

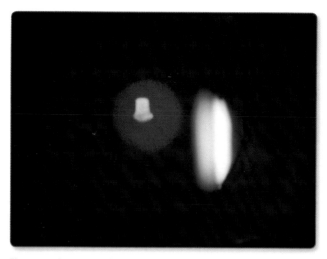

Figure 9.4 A posterior subcapsular cataract. (Courtesy of the medical photography department, Princess Alexandra Eye Pavilion, Edinburgh).

Management

Anaesthesia

The most common type of anaesthesia is an amide such as lidocaine 2% injected under the Tenon's capsule (fascial sheath of the eyeball) with a blunt curved needle (**Figure 9.5**). This anaesthetises the eye, paralyses the eye muscles and also temporarily blinds the patient as the optic nerve is affected. Variations include a retrobulbar or peribulbar injection with a sharp needle to paralyse the eye completely or topical drop anaesthesia in which only anaesthesia is achieved. The patient's eyelids are then thoroughly cleaned with iodinated fluid and a sterile drape is applied.

Positioning is important; the patient must be able to lie still as the procedure is performed under microscopy. General anaesthesia is rarely required, e.g. when positioning cannot be achieved or because of other patient factors.

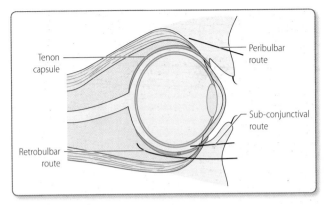

Figure 9.5 Periocular routes of drug administration.

Techniques

Phacoemulsification is the most common technique in the developed world; its use in poorer countries is limited by cost. Manual extracapsular cataract extraction is more common in developing countries and is also used for difficult operations in developed countries.

Phacoemulsification and extracapsular cataract extraction
Although there are variations in technique, but usually include the following:
· a 3-mm self-sealing incision is made to allow a phacoemulsifying probe into the eye
· a second smaller incision is made to allow a second assisting instrument into the eye
· a circular incision in the front of the lens capsule allows access to the cataractous lens
· the probe is inserted into the eye and all cataractous lens material is removed
· a foldable artificial lens is inserted, usually with the help of an introducing device, into the capsule
The wounds are usually self-sealing.

Phacoemulsification mechanism Fluid travels down the outside of the probe to keep the anterior chamber filled. The probe vibrates, causing an ultrasonic shockwave to be spread in front of it. This emulsifies the lens, which is then sucked through the central shaft (**Figure 9.6**).

In children, a similar technique is used, but, owing to a soft lens, the lens can easily be aspirated rather than expressed out, and absorbable sutures are often used to seal wounds.

Manual extracapsular cataract extraction This technique involves the following steps:

- a large incision is made, usually in the sclera or at the limbus
- a large opening is fashioned in the anterior capsule
- a special lens glide is then inserted under the lens to extract the lens
- a rigid artificial lens is placed into the capsule

The incision is closed with sutures if it is large or allowed to seal if it is small and self-sealing.

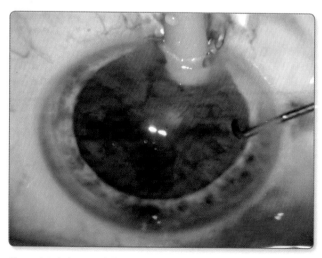

Figure 9.6 A phacoemulsification probe.

Recovery of vision is usually longer with this procedure, with sutures removed at approximately 3 months.

Intraocular lenses

Perhaps some of the biggest recent developments have been made in lens technology. The available types of intraocular lenses include rigid polymethylmethacrylate, flexible silicone and hydrophobic or hydrophilic acrylate. Newer lenses allow accommodation and correct for astigmatism.

Complications

Complications occur in <1% of operations. The posterior capsule can be ruptured, allowing the vitreous to prolapse and risking retinal detachment and macular oedema. After surgery, the greatest risk is endophthalmitis. This is usually an aggressive sight-threatening infection of the eye requiring antibiotics and often surgery.

Follow-up

Antibiotics (e.g. cefuroxime) are injected into the eye at the time of the operation. Usually, patients are discharged on the day of surgery and given regular topical antibiotics (e.g. chloramphenicol ointment for 1 week) and corticosteroid (e.g. dexamethasone for up to 4 weeks). Follow-up usually takes place in the week after surgery to ensure recovery is progressing as planned. Approximately 4 weeks after the phacoemulsification operation, patients can go to their optometrists to obtain glasses for full refractive correction.

Uvea

Uveitis – inflammation of the uvea – is an important cause of morbidity and loss of vision in ophthalmology; however, it continues to be relatively rarely seen in ophthalmic practice. The condition is often systemic and may require multispecialty follow-up for ongoing care and treatment.

Anatomy

The **uvea** is composed of the iris anteriorly and the choroid posteriorly, meeting at the ciliary body (**Figure 10.1**). The tissue is composed of a unique combination of vascular pigmented elements sandwiched between the sclera and retina. The choroid provides nutrition via arteries, and waste produced by retinal function is removed by choroidal veins. The juxtaposition of the choroid and retina exposes the potential for both inflammation and infection originating from the blood supply of neighbouring vascular beds.

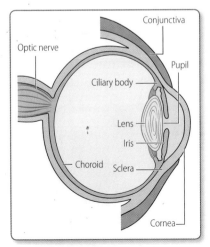

Figure 10.1 The uvea.

10.1 Clinical scenario

Photophobia

Presentation

A 35-year-old man presents to his GP with an ache in his right eye that becomes severe with light.

Diagnostic approach

The patient describes photophobia. There are very few causes of photophobia and therefore this is a helpful symptom to start the diagnosis. Careful questioning about associated symptoms should help narrow down the diagnosis further to help examination.

Differential diagnoses: For a summary of the causes of photophobia, see **Table 10.1**.

Further history

The patient's symptoms have gradually progressed over the last 2 days. The eye has become red and the vision has reduced slightly. There is no foreign body sensation and the eye only waters in bright light. The other eye is fine and he does not complain of any headache, fever or neck symptoms. However,

Unilateral/bilateral	Anatomical location	Associated symptoms
Unilateral	Corneal: abrasion, foreign body, keratitis	Foreign body sensation, sharp pain, watering
	Uveal: anterior, intermediate and posterior uveitis	Red eye, constant ache
Bilateral	Neurological: migraine, meningitis	Migraine: haloes before, headache and post-event photophobia Meningitis: neck stiffness, headache, rash, feverish
	Ophthalmic: bilateral uveitis	Red eye, constant ache

Table 10.1 Causes of photophobia

the patient has lower back pain, which is worse in the morning and improves on exercise.

Previous ocular history: The patient has had previous episodes of red eye that were similar to the current episode. These required treatment by an ophthalmologist.

Medications: The patient takes ibuprofen for back pain.

Diagnostic approach

The patient describes episodes of unilateral pain. The episodes are probably recurrent in view of the previous ocular history.

Examination

On examination, the patient is afebrile and systemically well with no rashes and no focal neurology or neck stiffness.

However, the patient is tender to palpation in the lower sacroiliac region; he has a kyphotic back posture and reduced anteroposterior flexion of the lumbar spine.

Ophthalmic examination: The ophthalmic examination is summarised in **Table 10.2**.

Diagnostic approach

The patient has a unilateral red eye without any external corneal pathology. Because of the patient's history of recurrent red eye and symptoms to indicate ankylosing spondylitis and sacroiliitis, the diagnosis is acute anterior uveitis.

10.2 Anterior uveitis

Anterior uveitis is inflammation of the anterior uveal tract, including the iris, ciliary body or both. It can be classified temporally into acute (<6 weeks) or chronic (>6 weeks). Causes can be infectious or non-infectious.

Epidemiology

Anterior uveitis is a relatively uncommon condition but presents regularly in ophthalmic practice because of frequent

	Right eye		Left eye
	Visual acuity	6/12	6/6
	Pupil	Normal direct and consensual reflex Pupil small	Normal direct and consensual reflex
	Conjunctiva	Perilimbal injection	White
	Cornea	Clear but small precipitates noted on cornea No foreign body or ulcer noted	Clear
	Anterior chamber	Hazy	Clear
	Lens	Pupil does not dilate well, leaving a hazy view of posterior segment	Clear and normal posterior segment

Table 10.2 Ophthalmic examination: results for a patient who presented with photophobia

recurrence. The incidence is approximately 12 per 100,000. There is no sex preponderance; however, the condition occurs more commonly in those aged over 20 years.

Causes

Most commonly (50–80% of cases), no cause of anterior uveitis is found despite thorough investigation. Human leukocyte antigen (HLA)-B27-related disease, which includes ankylosing spondylitis, is the next most common (20–50% of cases). Many causes of posterior uveitis may also present initially with an anterior uveitis. The most common causes of anterior uveitis are shown in **Table 10.3**.

Pathogenesis

The exact pathogenesis is still unknown. An unknown antigen is thought to provoke an inflammatory response that results in the breakdown of the eye–blood barrier. This breakdown enables white blood cells and protein to enter the anterior chamber.

Type	Causes
Idiopathic	—
Inflammatory	HLA-B27-related disease Sarcoidosis Behçet disease Kawasaki disease (mucocutaneous lymph node syndrome) Inflammatory bowel disease
Infectious	Bacterial: spirochaetes, *Borrelia burgdorferi* Parasitic: *Toxoplasma* Viral: herpetic disease

Table 10.3 Causes of acute anterior uveitis. HLA, human leukocyte antigen.

Clinical features

Patients have varying levels of photophobia, reduced vision and red eye. Examination reveals reduced vision and, occasionally, raised intraocular pressure. The pupil may be unreactive to light and miosed owing to posterior synechiae, i.e. inflammatory attachments between the lens capsule and iris (**Figure 10.2**). There is classically a perilimbal injection and the eye is tender to touch. If possible, the back of the eye should also be examined following dilation to exclude posterior uveitis.

The following general checklist is useful to rule out systemic disease. Does the patient have:
- Back pain (ankylosing spondylitis)?
- Rashes/tick bites (Lyme disease: *Borrellia burgdorferi* infection)?
- Breathing problems (tuberculosis, sarcoidosis)?
- Blood in the stool (inflammatory bowel disease)?
- Rash around eye (herpetic disease)?

Investigations

Because the majority of cases are idiopathic and non-recurrent, first cases of acute anterior uveitis are generally not investigated. However, recurrent and bilateral cases and those with features

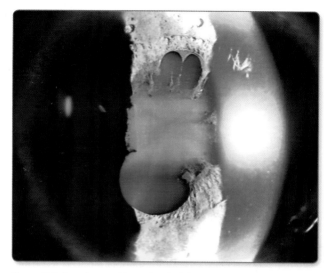

Figure 10.2 Posterior synechiae and perilimbal injection in acute anterior uveitis.

of systemic disease should be investigated with screening blood tests and a chest radiograph.

Differential diagnosis
Differential diagnoses may include any other cause for a red eye:
- *scleritis*: there is little photophobia, and the injection is not limited to the perilimbal area
- *conjunctivitis*: there is discharge from the eye, little photophobia, and the injection is usually throughout the conjunctiva
- *keratitis*: the cornea stains with fluorescein

Management
The aims of treatment are to reduce pain, treat inflammation and reduce the risk of complications. Acute anterior uveitis is usually treated with a strong topical corticosteroid such as dexamethasone or prednisolone given frequently – often hourly initially. Additionally, a dilating agent that is cycloplegic (i.e.

paralyses the accommodation reflex), such as cyclopentolate, is given to reduce pain and to break posterior synechiae.

Occasionally, if there is severe inflammation or marked synechiae that cannot be broken down, a subconjunctival injection is given containing dilating agents and a longer term corticosteroid (e.g. subconjunctival betamethasone). Following review, the treatment is then stepped down over several weeks in order to prevent recurrence. Chronic cases often require long-term corticosteroid and occasionally systemic treatment. Any systemic disease should also be treated and may require follow-up from other specialties.

Prognosis

The prognosis is generally very good, although recurrence is relatively common. This varies markedly from person to person. Complications include **posterior synechiae**, i.e. inflammatory membranes between the iris and the lens, which increase the risk of angle closure glaucoma. In addition, inflammation and corticosteroid treatment increase cataract formation and glaucoma risk.

10.3 Posterior uveitis and intermediate uveitis

Posterior uveitis is a term describing inflammation of the choroid and retina. Intermediate uveitis describes inflammation primarily in the posterior ciliary body; however, the term covers a broad range of diseases. These are anatomical classifications; clinically, there is usually marked overlap, occasionally resulting in a pan-uveitis that includes anterior uveitis as a feature.

Epidemiology

Posterior uveitis and intermediate uveitis are relatively rare conditions.

Causes

There are many causes of posterior uveitis. The common causes of posterior and intermediate uveitis are shown in **Table 10.4.**

Type	Causes
Infectious	Bacterial: syphilis, Lyme disease Viral: herpes simplex, herpes zoster, cytomegalovirus Fungal: *Candida* Parasitic: ***Toxoplasma***, toxocariasis
Non-infectious	Behçet disease Sarcoidosis Sympathetic ophthalma Vogt–Koyanagi–Harada syndrome (oculo-cutaneous syndrome) White dot syndrome Pars planitis

Table 10.4 Causes of posterior uveitis

The important area of differentiation, clinically, is whether the cause is infectious or non-infectious: commonly used immunosuppression treatment used in non-infectious uveitis may exacerbate infectious uveitis.

Pathogenesis

Although the exact pathogenesis is not known, animal models have highlighted several potential antigens in the eye. The body develops activated T cells that are thought to transmigrate through the retinal blood vessels. This is an appropriate response in infectious uveitis, but is inappropriate to unknown triggering antigens in non-infectious uveitis. The T cells assist in recruitment of further inflammatory cells, which lead to tissue destruction and the clinical features seen in uveitis.

Clinical features

Presentation is varied. Some patient's may have a painless blurring of vision whereas others have a hot, inflamed and red eye. Other symptoms include floaters and scotomas (i.e. areas of reduced vision surrounded by normal vision and metamorphopsias).

Examination often reveals reduced vision, from either vitritis or a macular retinal lesion. In pan-uveitis, signs may be similar to those in anterior uveitis. Fundoscopy is cloudy owing to vitritis, except in white dot syndromes and early retinitis and vasculitis (**Figure 10.3**). Retinitis appears with ill-defined white retinal lesions and haemorrhages. Choroiditis displays whitened lesions that heal with pigmentation (**Figure 10.4**). The most common causes of posterior uveitis are shown in **Table 10.5**. A full history, asking about systemic features of disease, is required, and systemic examination, especially of the skin and nails and respiratory system, should be made.

Investigations

Many of the causes of uveitis have a similar phenotype; therefore, investigative screens are important to look for disease, e.g. general blood tests such as full blood count and erythrocyte sedimentation rate. More specific tests include antinuclear antibody, Venereal Disease Research Laboratory and purified protein derivative tests and Lyme serology. A chest radiograph can be used to diagnose tuberculosis or sarcoidosis.

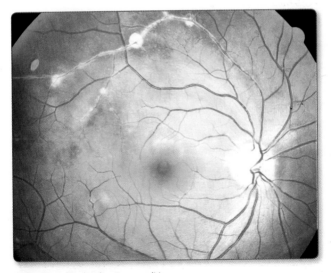

Figure 10.3 Fundus showing vasculitis

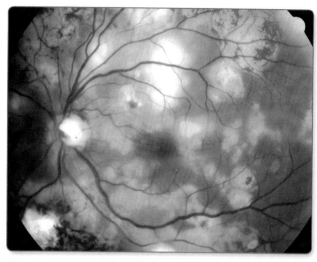

Figure 10.4 Fundus showing choroiditis.

Type	Causes
Intermediate	Multiple scleritis
Focal retinitis	Tuberculosis
Focal choroiditis	Tuberculosis Toxocara
Multifocal retinitis	Sarcoid Syphilis *Candida* Herpes simplex, varicella zoster, cytomegalovirus
Multifocal choroiditis	Sympathetic ophthalmic disease Histoplasma Sarcoid
Pan-uveitis	Infective endophthalmitis Behçet disease Sarcoid Syphilis

Table 10.5 Common causes of posterior uveitis

Differential diagnosis

For the differential diagnoses, see **Figure 3.1**.

Management

Urgent referral to an ophthalmic specialist is required to prevent or treat sight-threatening pathology. Usually, treatment initially includes topical corticosteroids such as dexamethasone, and a topical cycloplegic agent, such as cyclopentolate. Infectious causes are treated with the relevant medication. Severe sight-threatening non-infectious uveitis and infectious uveitis are usually treated initially with an oral corticosteroid such as prednisolone.

Chronic non-infectious uveitis may require non-steroid-based immunosuppression. This includes antimetabolites, such as azathioprine and methotrexate; alkylating agents, such as chlorambucil; antibiotics, such as ciclosporin or interferon; and newer biological treatments, such as infliximab.

Prognosis

Unlike anterior uveitis, the risk of vision loss is far greater with the posterior forms of uveitis. This may occur in up to 10% of cases.

Retinal disease

Retinal disease is relatively common and continues to increase in incidence and prevalence owing to an ageing population. The neural retina is highly dependent on its blood supply. It is affected by systemic causes of small blood vessel disease such as diabetes and hypertension. Retinal disease can often lead to permanent blindness. The field is becoming highly relevant with a range of new therapies being developed, including antineovascular therapy, gene therapy, transplantation and retinal implantation.

Anatomy and physiology

Beginning from the outside, the retina is made up of the choroid and the Bruch's membrane (latin name: lamina basalis choroideae), which is found below the **retinal pigment epithelium** (RPE) and neuroretina (**Figure 11.1**). At the innermost aspect of the **choroid** is the **choriocapillaris**, a fine latticework of fenestrated vessels that lies adjacent to the **Bruch's membrane**, which is a thin basement structure composed mainly of collagen.

The Bruch's membrane supports the RPE, a pigmented polygonal monolayer of cells. The RPE has microvilli on its inner surface that interdigitate with retinal photoreceptor outer segments. The RPE plays an important role in recycling of photoreceptor pigments, allowing the photoreceptors to continue functioning in transducing incoming light into electrical impulses.

Balanced on the photoreceptors is the neural retina, whose pyramid-like cellular structure has integrated processing power. A fluid-free extracellular environment is maintained in the neuroretina despite close proximity to the retinal and choroidal blood vessels by an inner and outer blood–retina barrier.

The transparency of the unmyelinated neuroretina allows light to pass through to the photoreceptors which are located on the outer aspect of the retina. The axons of the nerve fibre

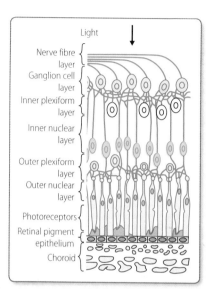

Figure 11.1 Retinal anatomy.

layer collect to exit the eyeball via the myelinated optic nerve, travelling back into the brain.

11.1 Clinical scenarios

Sudden loss of vision

Presentation

A 40-year-old man presents to the emergency department with sudden-onset, complete, painless loss of vision in the right eye.

Diagnostic approach

Loss of vision has a number of differential diagnoses. The further history can be used to ask more directed questions about the symptoms relating to the differential diagnoses (see Figure 3.2).

The patient describes sudden, unilateral and painless loss of vision. In sudden reduction of vision, the main differential diagnoses are vascular or haemorrhagic.

Further history

The patient feels that his vision is completely reduced in the right eye and he first noticed it that morning while cleaning the house. There were no flashing lights or floaters before the occurrence and there is no history of trauma. The patient does not complain of any temporal headache, fever or jaw claudication. There has been no change or return in the vision.

Previous medical history: The patient was diagnosed with type 1 diabetes 20 years ago. His glycated haemoglobin is recorded as 10.2. He also has hypertension and early diabetic nephropathy.

Medications: The patient injects subcutaneous insulin lispro (fast acting) three times a day, with insulin glargine (long acting) at night.

Diagnostic approach

The fact that the patient has poorly controlled type 1 diabetes strongly indicates possible vitreous haemorrhage secondary to new vessels or tractional retinal detachment, two of the ocular sequelae of poorly controlled diabetes. The dilated examination of the eye will give a clue to this. It is also important to examine the non-affected eye for clues to diabetic retinopathy and possible risk in the other eye.

Clinical insight

If the view on one eye is not clear always examine the opposite eye for clues about disease.

Examination

Ophthalmic examination:

Figure 11.2 shows the patient's retina; **Table 11.1** su mmarises the ophthalmic examination.

Diagnostic approach

The examination is important, revealing a normal relative afferent pupillary defect (RAPD). This helps rule out total retinal detachment, central retinal artery occlusion, marked central retinal vein occlusion and arteriopathic optic neuropathy.

The dilated fundus examination reveals no obvious view of the fundus, indicating a vitreous pathology on the right.

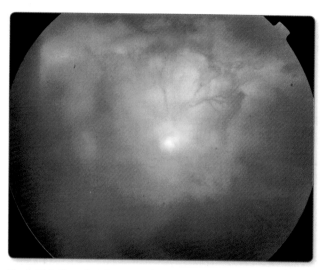

Figure 11.2 The retina of a patient who presented with sudden loss of vision.

Right eye		Left eye
Perception of light Able to note light projected to fundus in all areas	**Visual acuity**	6/6
Normal direct and consensual reflex	**Pupil**	Normal direct and consensual reflex
Clear	**Cornea**	Clear
Clear	**Anterior chamber**	Clear
Clear	**Lens**	Clear
Hazy	**Vitreous**	Clear
No clear view of fundus	**Fundus**	Clear view of fundus Reveals severe diabetic retinopathy and new vessels

Table 11.1 Ophthalmic examination: results for a patient who presented with sudden loss of vision

The left eye fundus examination shows marked diabetic changes indicative of severe diabetic retinopathy. This is further indication of vitreous haemorrhage secondary to diabetic new vessels.

Gradual loss of vision

Presentation
A 60-year-old man presents to the emergency department with a 2-day history of a shadow in his left eye.

Diagnostic approach
It is important to ascertain the characteristics of the 'shadow' more precisely. For instance, a mobile shadow that seems to be like a fly in the field of vision is more likely to have vitreous involvement, such as posterior vitreous detachment or a small vitreous haemorrhage. A fixed shadow is more likely to involve the retina, such as in a branch retinal artery occlusion, branch retinal vein occlusion and retinal detachment. Another differential diagnosis for a fixed shadow is optic nerve involvement, such as in glaucoma, optic nerve compression or optic neuritis.

The patient states that his vision is deteriorating rapidly. The cause is unlikely to be a vascular problem, such as arterial or venous occlusions, as these are usually immediate in effect. The patient is in the age range for all the conditions except optic neuritis, which most commonly affects those between 20 and 50 years of age.

The 2-day history makes it highly unlikely that this is a glaucomatous phenomenon. Chronic open angle glaucoma is usually a more slowly progressive phenomenon, occurring over months to years.

Further history
The patient says that the visual deterioration is fixed, with a greying in the field of vision that is now encroaching on the central vision. The shadow was preceded by intense flashing lights in the left eye and many small floaters.

Previous ocular history: The patient has marked myopia and wears varifocal glasses.

Diagnostic approach

The patient describes photopsia (i.e. flashing lights) and floaters. These are classic signs of **posterior vitreous detachment** (i.e. the detachment of the posterior vitreous face from the retina) or early retinal detachment. However, the fixed area of visual loss is not in keeping with a posterior vitreous detachment alone. The likelihood of retinal detachment is greatly increased by the patient having a marked myopia. The dilated examination should help to identify pathologies of the vitreous and retina.

Examination

Figure 11.3 shows the patient's retina (see also **Figure 3.2**).

Ophthalmic examination: Table 11.2 summarises the ophthalmic examination.

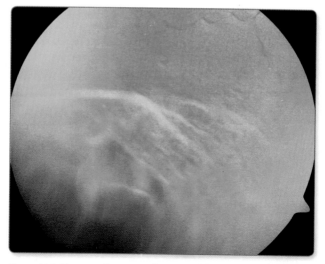

Figure 11.3 The retina of a patient who presented with gradual loss of vision.

Right eye		Left eye
6/6	**Visual acuity**	6/6
Normal direct and consensual reflex	**Pupil**	Normal direct and consensual reflex
Clear	**Cornea**	Clear
Clear	**Anterior chamber**	Clear
Clear	**Lens**	Clear
Clear	**Vitreous**	Large vitreous floater
Clear view of fundus	**Fundus**	Clear view of fundus Fundus has raised, white, wrinkled area with obvious tear
Normal vessels and disc	**Disc**	Normal vessels and disc

Table 11.2 Ophthalmic examination: results for a patient who presented with gradual loss of vision

Diagnostic approach

The examination reveals a retinal detachment with a tear most likely secondary to a posterior vitreous detachment occurring at the time the patient saw the flashing lights and floaters.

Clinical insight

Central vision can be normal until the retinal detachment crosses the macula. The aim is to diagnose the detachment before this occurs to preserve central vision.

11.2 Diabetic retinopathy

Diabetic retinopathy is a chronic disease affecting the retina in patients with long-standing diabetes.

Epidemiology

Diabetic retinopathy is steadily increasing in prevalence and is currently the most common cause of blindness in the working population. The increase in retinopathy is due to the overall increase in the prevalence of diabetes. Worldwide, there were 170 million cases in 2000, which is set to double by 2030.

Causes

Within 5 years of diagnosis, 25% of those with type 1 diabetes, 40% of those with type 2 diabetes on insulin and approximately 25% of those with type 2 diabetes on non-insulin treatment develop some form of retinopathy.

Pathogenesis

Poor glycaemic control leads to the death of the pericytes that surround small vessels and capillaries. Together these changes lead to vessel leakage and oedema. In addition, there is thickening of the basement membrane and vessel occlusion, leading to ischaemia. Ischaemia leads to release of factors, including vascular endothelial growth factor, which increases oedema and new vessel formation. These fragile new vessels often bleed, resulting in vitreous haemorrhage. The resultant resolution with scarring leads to retinal traction and can result in retinal detachment.

Clinical features

In countries with an annual diabetic eye examination, the majority of newly diagnosed patients are asymptomatic. Others patients with diabetic retinopathy may have varying symptoms according to the type and severity of retinopathy. Generally, the most common symptom is a gradual painless reduction in vision in diabetic macular oedema. Those with a vitreous haemorrhage have a more sudden painless loss of vision from bleeding new vessels.

On examination, a patient with diabetes may have various retinal changes. These are fully described below.

Patients with diabetes commonly also have a poor tear film, cataracts and may have ocular motility abnormalities owing to occlusion of small blood vessels to the rectus muscles.

Diagnostic criteria

Diagnosing diabetic retinal disease is divided into grading macular area disease and more generalised retinal disease, which is often called background diabetic retinopathy. Several criteria exist, all correlating disease severity to the risk of visual loss.

Early diabetic retinopathy (*Figure 11.4*): Early diabetic retinopathy is signified by dot haemorrhages and blot haemorrhages. In addition, there may be yellowish exudates and cotton wool spots, which are pale fluffy areas.

Preproliferative retinopathy (*Figure 11.5*): Preproliferative retinopathy is a more severe form of early disease with changes throughout the retina.

The Early Treatment of Diabetic Retinopathy Study suggested that preproliferative retinopathy was shown by blot haemorrhages in all four quadrants, venous beading in two quadrants and any intraretinal microvascular anomalies, which appear as small vascular bundles in the retina often away from major blood vessels.

Proliferative diabetic retinopathy (*Figure 11.6*): Proliferative diabetic retinopathy is retinal disease with formation of any new vessels.

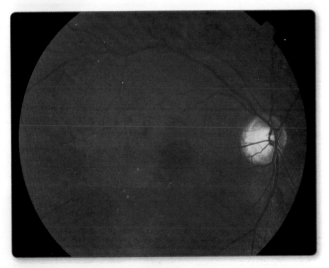

Figure 11.4 Early diabetic retinopathy.

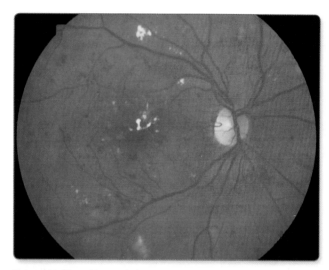

Figure 11.5 Preproliferative diabetic retinopathy.

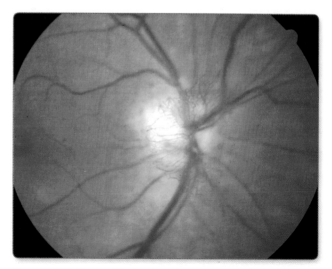

Figure 11.6 Proliferative diabetic retinopathy.

Diabetic maculopathy (*Figure 11.7*): Maculopathy is diabetic disease of the macula. In terms of diabetic disease, this is defined by an area of approximately one disc diameter around the fovea. Maculopathy can include any form of haemorrhage or exudate. However, oedema in this region can lead to severe reduction in central vision.

Investigations

Ocular coherence tomography (OCT) is increasingly used to monitor macular oedema. Fluorescein angiography is used to help diagnose new vessels, quantify chronic changes and define areas of macular oedema prior to treatment. In cases when central vision deteriorates with no obvious cause, it can be used to show loss of capillary perfusion to the macula in ischaemic maculopathy.

Differential diagnosis

Early diabetic retinopathy with blot haemorrhages can be mistaken for other causes of vessel disease. These include

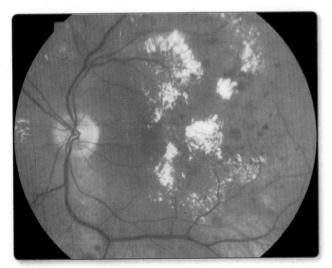

Figure 11.7 Diabetic maculopathy.

retinal vein occlusion, carotid artery occlusion and radiation retinopathy.

Management

Management of diabetic retinopathy varies as to the severity of disease.

The ideal management is prevention. Patients should be assessed for the effectiveness of prevention at clinic visits. This includes glycaemic control and monitoring blood pressure. Discussion with patients and their diabetic clinicians can sometimes help to prevent complications later.

Background diabetic retinopathy

Background diabetic retinopathy is monitored on a 6-monthly to annual basis with screening.

Preproliferative retinopathy

Preproliferative retinopathy is monitored in the clinic on a 4- to 6-monthly basis. Depending on patient factors, such as compliance with treatment, patients can be treated with peripheral panretinal laser.

> ### Clinical insight
>
> Initially peripheral panretinal laser treatment consists of 2400–3000 laser burns; which induce regression of new vessels. This technique sacrifices the peripheral retina in order to preserve overall vision.

> ### Clinical insight
>
> Although the mechanism is poorly understood, laser treatment for macular oedema is thought to modify the localised inflammatory response, leading to absorption of fluid and hence prevention of further worsening of vision. However, the low-level laser itself does lead to some loss of photoreceptors.

Proliferative diabetic retinopathy with haemorrhage

Vitreous haemorrhage is cleared with a **vitrectomy**, an intraocular surgical procedure used to extract the vitreous.

Diabetic macular oedema

Diabetic macular oedema is treated by very low-power laser to areas of oedema.

Prognosis

The prognosis generally depends on the patient. It is good for those who regularly attend for review, have good glycaemic control and maintain low blood pressures.

11.3 Hypertensive retinopathy

Hypertension is a systemic disease. There are a large variety of manifestations of retinal damage, which can correlate with other end-organ damage.

Epidemiology

The risk of hypertensive retinopathy increases with hypertension. The prevalence has been reported to be between 2% and 15% depending on the population studied. The prevalence of hypertensive retinopathy, like systemic hypertension, is higher among the Afro-Caribbean population and in those over the age of 40.

Pathogenesis

Retinal arterioles are similar to those found in the brain. They have no internal elastic lamina or continuous muscular coat, but they do have tight junctions. Choroidal vessels are fenestrated to enable passage of substances to the RPE and outer retina. The prime mechanism for control is autoregulation of flow by arteriolar constriction. Early hypertension results in diffuse constriction of retinal vessels. This can become persistent, leading to thickening with focal constriction. Later, breaking of tight junctions leads to microaneurysms, macroaneurysms, haemorrhages, hard exudates and cotton wool spots.

Clinical features

Patients rarely have visual disturbance unless they have haemorrhage. More often, patients are noted to have retinal changes on a routine visit to the optometrist. Examination by fundoscopy can reveal diffuse or focal vessel narrowing, microaneurysms, macroaneurysms, cotton wool spots, exudates and disc swelling.

Associated features may include retinal vein occlusions and vitreous haemorrhages.

Diagnostic criteria

The Scheie classification is used for staging hypertensive retinopathy (**Table 11.3**). It also grades the light reflex changes that occur as a result of arteriolosclerotic changes in hypertensive retinopathy (**Table 11.4**).

Investigations

Blood pressure should be monitored. In addition, where applicable, investigations should be made in accordance with systemic findings. Moderate retinal findings should also prompt

Stage	Description
0	Diagnosis of hypertension but no visible retinal abnormalities
1	Diffuse arteriolar narrowing, but no focal constriction
2	More pronounced arteriolar narrowing with focal constriction
3	Focal and diffuse narrowing, with retinal haemorrhage
4	Retinal oedema, hard exudates and optic disc oedema

Table 11.3 Scheie classification for staging hypertensive retinopathy (Scheie HG. AMA Arch Ophthalmol 1953;49:117–38)

Grade	Description
0	Normal
1	Broadening of the light reflex with minimal arteriolovenous compression
2	Light reflex changes and crossing changes more prominent
3	Copper-wire appearance, with more prominent arteriolovenous compression
4	Silver-wire appearance, with severe arteriovenous crossing changes

Table 11.4 Scheie classification for grading light reflex changes in hypertensive retinopathy (Scheie HG. AMA Arch Ophthalmol 1953;49:117–38)

investigation of other end-organs, including renal function and cardiovascular risk.

Differential diagnosis

The differential diagnoses for hypertensive retinopathy include:

- *diabetic retinopathy*: there is a history of diabetes, with more blot haemorrhages
- *retinal vein occlusion*: there are streaked haemorrhages in the region of the vessels
- *papilloedema*: usually, there are purely disc changes or changes around the disc

Management

Retinopathy changes usually reverse once blood pressure control returns to normal. Therefore, the aim is to stabilise systemic blood pressure. This is performed with lifestyle changes and medication as required. The retina can be reviewed in severe retinopathy by an ophthalmologist.

Stage 4 changes indicate malignant hypertension and warrant immediate medical referral.

Prognosis

The majority of ocular changes are reversible unless vein occlusion occurs. The greater concern is the risk of cardiac and cerebrovascular disease. The risk of stroke is two or three times higher in those with retinopathy, whereas the risk of cardiovascular events is doubled with retinopathy.

11.4 Retinal vein occlusion

Retinal vein occlusion is a blockage of retinal veins. If the blockage occurs before the vein enters the optic nerve, this results in a branch or hemispheric vein occlusion. If the blockage occurs after the retinal veins have entered the optic nerve, this usually results in a central retinal venous occlusion affecting the whole of the retina.

Epidemiology

Retinal vein occlusions are relatively common, with a prevalence of between 1% and 2% in those over 40 years. Branch retinal venous occlusions are approximately four times more common than central vein occlusions.

Causes

For the causes of retinal vein occlusion, see **Table 11.5**.

Pathogenesis

As in venous occlusion elsewhere in the body, this results from alterations to Virchow's triad: haemodynamic changes, vessel damage and hypercoagulability. Most commonly in branch retinal vein occlusion, this results from reduced flow at arterial cross-over points. Consequently, hypertension is a risk factor.

Clinical features

Patients commonly report a sudden, painless, unilateral reduction of vision in branch retinal vein occlusion (**Figure 11.8**) and central retinal vein occlusion (**Figure 11.9**). Depending on whether the macula is involved, vision will be reduced on testing.

Branch retinal vein occlusion	Central retinal vein occlusion
Systemic hypertension	Elevated intraocular pressure
Diabetes mellitus	Systemic hypertension
Renal disease	Diabetes mellitus
Hyperlipidaemia	Renal disease
Homocystinuria	Hyperlipidaemia
Anticardiolipin antibodies	Homocystinuria
	Anticardiolipin antibodies
	Inflammatory eye disease, e.g. Behçet uveitis

Table 11.5 Diseases that increase the risk of retinal vein occlusion

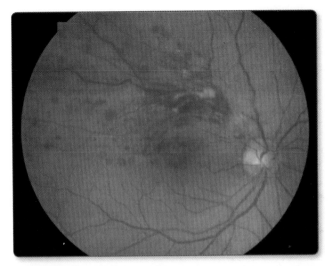

Figure 11.8 A branch retinal vein occlusion.

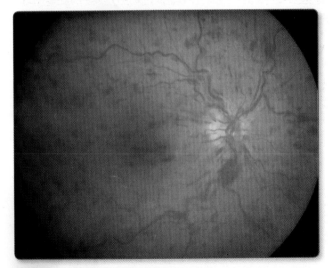

Figure 11.9 A central retinal vein occlusion.

Fundus examination reveals:

- haemorrhages
- cotton wool spots
- exudates
- tortuous vessels

Generally, the more ischaemic the central retinal vein occlusion, the more signs are apparent and the lower the vision. A RAPD indicates the likelihood of ischaemia.

In late presentations, new vessels, prompted by intraocular ischaemia, may be visible on the iris and there may be high pressure as these vessels block the trabecular meshwork.

Investigations

The patient's blood pressure should be checked along with simple blood tests, including full blood count, fasting cholesterol and glucose. In those under 50, a coagulation screen may be performed.

OCT and a fluorescein angiogram are often used to assess macular involvement and the amount of ischaemia, and hence the risk of neovascularisation.

Differential diagnosis

The differential diagnoses for retinal vein occlusion include:

- *diabetic retinopathy*: a history of diabetes and usually more generalised blots and hard exudates
- *hypertensive retinopathy*: localised vessel occlusion, usually with more flame haemorrhages

Management

In order to reduce the risk of further occlusions, cardiovascular risk factors should be modified, especially if the patient is hypertensive. If there is a high risk of new vessel formation or actual neovascularisation, laser photocoagulation is used to treat the area of affected retina. Increasingly, antivascular endothelial growth factor drugs are used to treat oedema and neovascularisation in retinal vein occlusion to help preserve vision. An intraocular glucocorticoid (dexamethasone implant) is sometimes used to treat persistent macular oedema in branch retinal vein occlusion.

Prognosis

The prognosis varies with the type of vein occlusion. Small, non-macula-involving branch vessel occlusions may not affect long-term vision at all. However, central retinal, macula-involving branch and ischaemic vein occlusions affecting large areas of retina may have a deep permanent visual deficit. Patients may also have long-term complications.

11.5 Retinal artery occlusion and amaurosis fugax

Retinal artery occlusion can be either central or branch artery occlusion. Central retinal artery occlusion results from a blockage anywhere from the origin of the artery, as the first branch of the ophthalmic artery, to its first branch, usually at the entry to the retina. **Amaurosis fugax** (from the Greek for darkness and the Latin for fleeting) describes the temporary reduction in vision that arises from temporary loss of circulation. These conditions are equivalent to strokes or transient ischaemic attacks in the cerebral circulation.

Epidemiology

Retinal artery occlusion has an incidence of approximately 1 per 100,000 per year and increases with age, peaking in the sixth and seventh decades. The central retinal artery is more commonly blocked than the branch retinal artery.

Causes

The causes of retinal artery occlusion are shown in **Table 11.6**.

Pathogenesis

The retinal artery is the first branch of the ophthalmic artery, which in turn is the first branch of the internal carotid artery. It supplies the inner part of the neuroretina. The choroid, RPE

Central retinal artery occlusion	Branch retinal artery occlusion	Amaurosis fugax
Embolism	Embolism	Embolism
Atherosclerotic disease	Vasospasm	Hydrostatic
Vasospasm		Vasospasm
Endarteritis, e.g. giant cell		

Table 11.6 Causes of arterial occlusions

and outer neuroretina are supplied by the ciliary arteries, which are a later branch of the ophthalmic artery.

Complete occlusion of the retina for about 2 hours is thought to lead to complete irreversible loss of vision, although in reality occlusion is rarely complete. At this point, the retina is pale and oedematous, and usually a 'cherry red spot' is observed at the macula from the exposed choroidal circulation at this thinner portion of the retina.

Clinical features

Patients with these conditions describe sudden-onset, painless reduction in vision. Always ask patients about cardiovascular risk factors.

In branch retinal artery occlusion, central vision may be spared. Amaurosis fugax typically lasts only seconds.

Patients with amaurosis fugax will have a normal ocular examination. In retinal artery occlusion, examination will reveal a reduction in central and peripheral vision in central retinal artery occlusion and an incomplete loss of central vision in macula-affecting occlusions of the branch retinal artery. Confrontation visual field testing helps to differentiate branch from central retinal occlusions, and an RAPD is more suggestive of a central retinal occlusion.

Fundoscopy may reveal an early whitening with oedema in the territory of the vessels affected with a cherry red spot if the macula is involved early on, although later there may be complete pallor as oedema progresses (**Figure 11.10**).

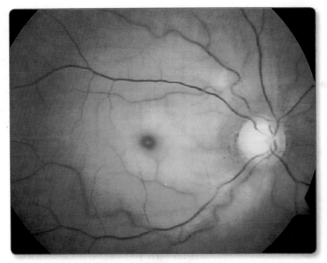

Figure 11.10 Central retinal artery occlusion with a cherry red macula.

Investigations

Systemic evaluation should include a full blood count, fasting glucose and cholesterol, erythrocyte sedimentation rate, C-reactive protein and a cardiac examination, looking for atrial fibrillation.

Patients should be referred to the local stroke team for further work-up of risks, including a carotid ultrasound and echocardiogram.

Differential diagnosis

Differential diagnoses include any cause of painless loss of vision (see **Figure 3.2**).

Management

Initial management should be prompt in order to restore circulation. There are a number of emergency treatments, most of which have only anecdotal evidence of success:

- inhaling a higher than normal level of carbon dioxide, e.g. by the patient breathing into a paper bag

- using topical glaucoma drops (e.g. timolol)
- ocular massage
- anterior chamber paracentesis, in which a temporary incision is made at the limbus; this can be performed by an ophthalmologist and can dramatically reduce intraocular pressure

Thrombolytics have not shown any benefit in recent trials.

Prognosis

The prognosis depends directly on the time taken to restore circulation. If there is complete circulation loss for longer than 6 hours, restoration of vision is unlikely. Attempts at restoration should still be made up to 24 hours after an event, in case there is only a partial occlusion.

11.6 Age-related macular degeneration

Age-related macular degeneration (ARMD), as its name suggests, is a degeneration that affects older patients and results in degenerative changes to the retina. There are two main types: dry and wet ARMD.

Epidemiology

ARMD is thought to affect up to 600,000 people in the UK, resulting in legal blindness in over 100,000. Although wet ARMD constitutes only 10–15% of cases of ARMD, it results in 80% of ARMD blind registrations.

The risk of blindness increases with age. The prevalence of advanced ARMD is approximately 1–2% in those over 40, but increases to over 7% in those over 75. There is a higher prevalence among white populations than among Afro-Caribbean or Asian populations.

Causes

ARMD is thought to be a complex disease with a variety of genetic and environmental factors. Recently, genome-wide scanning has identified a wide variety of genes. Many are related to the alternative complement pathway. Other risks include smoking, hypertension, obesity and low dietary antioxidants such as zinc.

Pathogenesis

The mechanism of disease is incompletely understood. It is thought that genetic predisposition increases the likelihood of localised inflammation at the back of the eye. This may be increased further by environmental factors such as smoking. This leads to subretinal deposition and the formation of drusen. Excess deposition and drusen may lead to damage to RPE cells, which, in turn, release inflammatory factors such as vascular endothelial growth factor. This incites new blood vessels that leak and lead to the wet ARMD features. In dry ARMD, RPE cell death leads to subsequent atrophy of photoreceptors.

Clinical features

Patients initially may not have any abnormalities. In dry degeneration, there is a gradual reduction in central vision. Wet ARMD will lead to a sudden-onset, painless distortion or loss of central vision. Dilated examination in early disease may show areas of yellow discrete lesions in the macula suggestive of drusen. In later disease, areas of atrophy are found in dry ARMD or haemorrhage and exudate in wet ARMD (**Figures 11.11** and **11.12**).

Investigations

The patient's other eye should be examined as there is a risk of bilateral disease. In wet ARMD, a fluorescein angiogram can be used to confirm the diagnosis by showing leaky retinal vessels under the macula. OCT can be used to follow the exudates.

Differential diagnosis

The differential diagnosis is diabetic maculopathy, in which patients have diabetes as well as blot haemorrhages and discrete exudates in the eye.

Management

Initial management should include focus on modifiable risk factors. This is especially true of dry ARMD, which has no

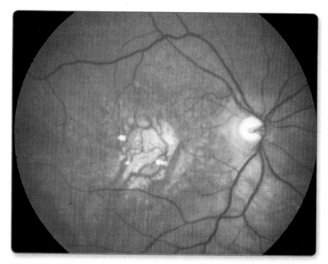

Figure 11.11 Dry age-related macular degeneration.

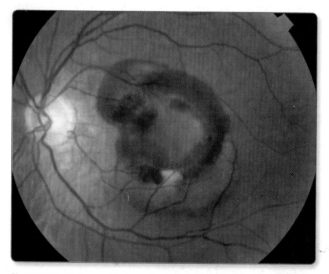

Figure 11.12 Wet age-related macular degeneration with macular haemorrhage and exudate.

definitive treatment. However, there is evidence that smoking cessation, weight and blood pressure control and increasing antioxidant and omega 3 fatty acid intake can reduce progression.

Wet ARMD is now treated with intravitreal antivascular endothelial growth factors as first-line treatment. These are initially given three times over 3 months and then whenever recurrences as signified by fluid visible on ocular coherence tomography. Less commonly, in certain types of wet ARMD, laser treatment is used.

Prognosis

New treatments have reduced the number of patients going blind from ARMD. However, almost half of those with advanced ARMD in one eye will go on to develop ARMD in the other eye within 5 years. Without treatment, 12% of those with blindness from wet ARMD in one eye will be blind in 5 years.

Wet ARMD vision can now be stabilised for at least 2 years and improved in one third of patients with antivascular endothelial growth factor treatments.

11.7 Retinal tears/detachment

Retinal detachment is the detachment of the neuroretina from the RPE. This section focuses on **rhegmatogenous retinal detachment** (rhegmatogenous is derived from the Greek word *rhegma*, meaning break), i.e. retinal detachment secondary to breaks in the retina.

Epidemiology

Approximately 15% of people have retinal breaks in their lifetime, but the annual incidence of retinal detachment is only 15 per 100,000. Frequency increases with age.

Causes

Risks include age, myopia, intraocular surgery, weaknesses in the retina such as lattice dystrophy, and genetic conditions such as Marfan syndrome.

Pathogenesis

Most commonly, rhegmatogenous retinal detachment occurs secondary to posterior vitreous detachment. With age, the collagen-rich, jelly-like vitreous becomes more water-like in its response to eye movement. Yet, it is still attached to the retina. This may eventually lead to the posterior vitreous detaching from the retina. If this detachment also results in a full-thickness retinal tear, the fluid in the vitreous can flow under the retina and cause the retina to detach. However, not all breaks lead to retinal detachment.

Clinical features

Most patients have unilateral floaters and about one quarter have flashing lights. Those who go on to have retinal detachment may eventually notice a gradually increasing shadow in one eye.

> **Guiding principle**
>
> Symptoms of posterior vitreous detachment, retinal tear and detachment may initially be very similar; hence, thorough examination is important to rule out tears or detachments.

Visual acuity with tears and detachments may be normal if the central retina is unaffected. However, vision deteriorates with macular involvement. Complete retinal detachment may lead to loss of the red reflex and a RAPD. Retinal detachment may be diagnosed with confrontation visual field testing. Fundoscopy reveals vitreous lined with brownish pigmented material, often called tobacco dust. The posterior vitreous attachment may be visible as a ring. Tears are usually visible in the periphery and most often superotemporally. Detachments give the retina a whitened appearance (**Figure 11.13**). Rarely, the view of the fundus is obscured owing to secondary vitreous haemorrhage.

Investigations

Ultrasound should be used to check retinal integrity in cases in which the retina is not visible.

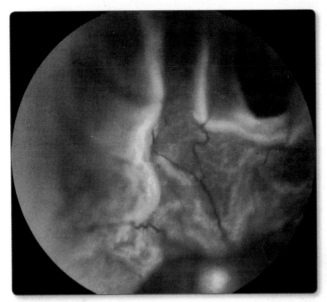

Figure 11.13 Retinal detachment.

Differential diagnosis

The differential diagnoses for retinal tears/detachment include:

- *serous retinal detachment*: usually there is a concave change, with no tear
- *retinoschisis*: this is a split in the retina; it is usually concave, bilateral and more common in hypermetropes
- *tractional retinal detachment*: the membranes are obvious; this is more common in patients with diabetes

Management

Posterior vitreous detachment

No treatment is required, but patients should be warned to return if new floaters, flashes or shadow are noticed as these are signs of a progression to retinal tear or detachment.

Tears

Tears can be treated with laser to the retina to surround the tear.

If there is some fluid or laser treatment is ineffective, external cryotherapy can be used to seal the break.

Retinal detachment

There are two main methods for treatment of retinal detachment. The most common is vitrectomy, which involves using small instruments in the eye to cut and suction the vitreous. Air is then used to force the subretinal fluid out and flatten the retina before laser or cryotherapy treatment is used to seal the hole. Finally, gas or silicone oil is left in the vitreous cavity to keep the retina flat.

Alternatively, a buckle or sponge can be sewn to the outside of the eye to indent the sclera and hence push on the retina and close the tear. Closure is assisted with cryotherapy.

Prognosis

The prognosis is good for tears and early retinal detachments. The visual prognosis is poor for macular involvement of more than a couple of days.

11.8 Retinitis pigmentosa

Retinitis pigmentosa (RP) describes a cluster of different inherited diseases that are linked by common symptomatology and signs.

Epidemiology

Approximately 1 in every 4000 people worldwide is thought to have RP. Half of the cases are autosomal recessive, one third autosomal dominant and approximately 15% are X-linked.

Pathogenesis

The common pathological pathway leads to photoreceptor death in RP. Causes can include abnormalities in photoreceptor metabolism and in the retinal pigment epithelium recycling of photoactive chemicals. Generally, the rods are the first to be lost, leading to mid-peripheral vision loss and dark-adapting abnormalities. Central vision decreases once the cones are involved. The death of cells can lead to a mild inflammation in the vitreous.

Clinical features

Presentation is variable depending on the type of retinitis. It is important to note that about one third of patients with RP have non-ocular findings in syndromic forms. Initially, patients usually have poor dark adaptation followed by night blindness. Visual field loss is initially mid-peripheral, followed by the far periphery, before finally losing central vision.

Examination may reveal early cataract and vitreous activity. The classic fundus appearance includes bone spicule pigmentation, a waxy-looking disc and attenuated blood vessels (**Figure 11.14**). Visual field loss may be found with confrontation visual field testing.

Patients should also be examined systemically for other syndromic types of RP.

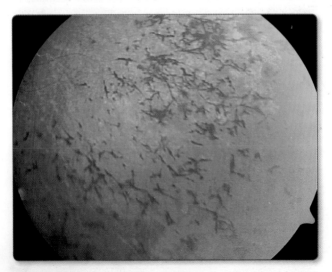

Figure 11.14 Classic bone spicule pigmentation in the mid-periphery of retinitis pigmentosa.

Diagnostic criteria

Some of the systemic associations of RP are summarised in **Table 11.7**.

Investigations

Patients should be investigated for potentially treatable forms and also syndromes that may harm general health. Serum phytane can be checked for Refsum disease (phytanic acid storage disease) and the lipid profile for abetalipoproteinaemia. Finally, an ECG can be performed to check for heart block in Kearns–Sayre disease (oculocraniosomatic disease).

Possible macular oedema may reduce vision rapidly; this can be checked with OCT or fluorescein angiography. Diagnosis can be helped by genetic testing and ocular electrophysiology looking for rod dysfunction.

Differential diagnosis

The differential diagnoses for RP include:

- *dry macular degeneration*: usually there is marked macular atrophy with little change elsewhere; in addition, the dark adaptation abnormality is less
- *drug toxicity*: usually due to hyroxychloroquine/chloroquine use
- *vitamin A deficiency*: this is caused by poor nutrition and can be seen as corneal and conjunctival white patches

Syndrome	Signs
Usher syndrome	Hearing loss
Kearns–Sayre disease	Ophthalmoplegia, heart block and ptosis
Abetalipoproteinaemia	Spinocerebellar degeneration, fat-soluble vitamin deficiency, malabsorption
Bardet–Biedl syndrome	Polydactyly, renal dysfunction and short stature

Table 11.7 Syndromic forms of retinitis pigmentosa

Management

Appropriate treatment should be given for treatable forms. This includes a phytane-free diet in Refsum disease and high-dose vitamin A in abetalipoproteinaemia.

Patients should be advised to reduce oxidative stress by, for instance, avoiding sunlight. High-dose vitamin A has also been found to reduce progression of the disease.

Acetazolamide can be used orally and topically to help in the treatment of acute-onset macular oedema during the disease course.

Prognosis

Most patients are legally blind by 40, with severity being greatest in those with X-linked disease. Progression occurs in all types of disease, although Refsum disease and abetalipoproteinaemia can be relatively well controlled. Consequently, counselling and early support with visual aids are important. This is especially true for patients with Usher syndrome, who also have severe hearing loss and require special education and assistance from childhood.

11.9 Adult retinal tumours

As with elsewhere in the body, retinal tumours can divided into either benign or malignant, and into primary or secondary. Primary retinal tumours are relatively rare. Different primary tumours derive from cells in the neuroretina, RPE and choroid. However, the choroid is a relatively common site for metastasis owing to its vascularity. Retinoblastoma, a primary tumour of the neuroretina, is discussed in Chapter 14.

Epidemiology

The epidemiology of retinal tumours varies as to the type of tumour. Generally, most primary tumours are rare; exceptions include choroidal naevus, which occurs in up to 10% of the population, and congenital hypertrophy of the RPE, which occurs in up to 1% of the population. Some of the common types of retinal tumour are listed in **Table 11.8**.

	Primary	Secondary
Benign	Choroidal naevus Choroidal haemangioma Choroidal osteoma Capillary haemangioma Cavernous haemangioma Astrocytoma Congenital hypertrophy of retinal pigment epithelium	
Malignant	Choroidal melanoma Lymphoma	Choroidal metastasis: the most common include lung, breast, bowel, kidney, skin Lymphoma

Table 11.8 Types of retinal tumour

Pathogenesis

The most commonly seen tumour is the choroidal naevus, which is a relatively flat, benign lesion (<2 mm). However, it may rarely convert to a choroidal malignant melanoma. Choroidal melanoma is graded in a similar way to skin melanomas, with size and depth being the prime factors related to prognosis. Small (<10 mm in diameter), medium (10–15 mm diameter) and large (>15 mm in diameter) choroidal melanomas have an increasingly worse prognosis. Certain cell types and genetic mutations also confer greater chance of progression.

Other tumours are related to systemic conditions (**Table 11.9**).

Clinical features

Patients may have painless, unilateral reduction in vision, especially if the macula and optic nerve are involved. Occasionally, they have flashing lights from retinal irritation. The previous medical history can help to diagnose systemic conditions. Examination may reveal a reduced visual acuity or field reduction on confrontation. Dilated fundoscopy usually reveals any abnormal pathology, with discoloration or alteration in the shape of the retina with raised lesions.

Tumour	Systemic disease relationship	Systemic features
Retinal haemangioma	von Hippel–Lindau syndrome	Haemangioblastomas of cerebellum, brain and spinal cord Phaeochromocytoma Renal cell carcinoma Visceral cysts
Astrocytoma	Tuberous sclerosis (neurofibromatosis type 1)	Ashleaf spots Shagreen patches Subungual fibroma Adenoma sebaceum Cerebral astrocytoma
Atypical congenital hypertrophic retinal pigment epithelium	Familial adenomatous polyposis	Multiple colonic polyps that transform to malignant adenocarcinoma

Table 11.9 Systemic associations of retinal tumours

Investigations

Retinal ultrasound is valuable in helping to differentiate a benign naevus from a malignant melanoma. Generally, thickness >2 mm and subretinal fluid are associated with choroidal melanoma, and thickness <1.5 mm and a flat retina are associated with a choroidal naevus. Oncologists can help in the investigation of other specific tumours.

Differential diagnosis

The most difficult differential diagnoses in adult retinal tumours are to differentiate between the tumours themselves. Other differential diagnoses include:

- *diabetic new vessels*: these may mimic haemangiomas; however, there are usually other retinal changes, and fluorescein will also show intraocular ischaemia
- *prominent vortex veins*: there are usually bilateral temporal veins entering under the retina

- *old ARMD*: usually there are central macular changes only, with changes in the opposite eye

Management

Management varies with the type of tumour. Benign tumours can usually be observed unless they cause visual disturbance. Choroidal naevi are usually observed on an annual basis by optometrists or ophthalmologists to monitor for malignant conversion. A photographic record is useful.

The Collaborative Ocular Melanoma Study indicated that small choroidal melanomas should be observed, whereas plaque radiotherapy is suggested for medium-sized tumours with enucleation suggested for large tumours.

Lymphomas require radiotherapy or intravitreal or systemic chemotherapy. Metastatic disease requires urgent liaison with oncology colleagues for staging and management.

Prognosis

The prognosis is usually good in most benign conditions, but worsens with size and invasion in choroidal melanomas. Both lymphoma and metastatic disease have a poor prognosis as eye manifestations are usually late-stage manifestations.

Optic nerve and visual pathways

The optic nerve and visual pathway relay information from the retina to the main visual processing centre in the occipital lobe. Although the pathway is composed of thousands of topographically organised nerves wrapped in myelin, its long course through the brain makes it susceptible to damage. The most common area for damage is the intraocular optic nerve, from diseases such as glaucoma. Damage to the pathway can lead to dense, irreversible and debilitating visual deficit.

Anatomy and physiology

Light is converted from photons to neural impulses by the photoreceptors. Rather interestingly, the light must travel through the transparent neuroretina to reach the photoreceptors underneath. This image is sent to the brain by a topographical network of nerves that have a partial crossover at the chiasm. This results in nasal fibres, which carry information from the temporal visual field, arriving at the contralateral midbrain (**Figure 12.1**).

The integration of visual information from each part of the visual field requires a precise orderly arrangement of nerve fibres relaying information to the main processing centre in the occipital lobe. This is called **retinotopic** organisation, and enables high-resolution, binocular stereo vision.

12.1 Clinical scenarios

Eye pain

Presentation

A 60-year-old woman presents to the emergency department with pain in her left eye.

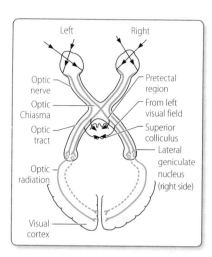

Figure 12.1 The visual pathway.

Diagnostic approach

Pain is a valuable clue to the possible location of abnormalities within the eye. It is important to characterise the kind of pain and to clarify any associated symptoms in order to help narrow down differential diagnoses.

Further history

The patient states that the pain has come on during the evening over the last couple of hours and is a severe ache around the eye, causing a headache. The patient feels that her vision has reduced. At the same time, the patient has become nauseous and has severe abdominal pain. **Table 12.1** lists the characteristics of pain according to anatomical location.

Previous ocular history: The patient is hypermetropic. Her last optician's examination revealed cataracts in both eyes.

Diagnostic approach

The patient describes a reduction in vision, nausea and a gradual onset of pain during the evening. With a patient who is hypermetropic, there is an increased risk of angle

Anatomical location	Pain characteristics	Associated symptoms
Lids	Burning if blepharitis Ache and tenderness to touch if orbital or preseptal cellulitis	Gritty sensation Orbital cellulitis: double vision, reduced vision, reduced colour vision
Conjunctiva	Burning sensation in conjunctivitis	Watering of eyes and marked redness. Viral symptoms may precede an eye condition
Sclera	Severe boring pain, keeping the patient up at night. Severe tenderness to palpation	Red eye Medical history may include connective tissue disorders
Cornea	Sharp knife-like pain with some photophobia	Tearing and foreign body sensation
Iris	Iritis results in an ache with marked photophobia increasing over hours to days	Hazy vision and red eye Previous occurrences common
Drainage angle blockage	Severe ache increasing over hours	Red eye Reduction in vision with haloes around lights and nausea

Table 12.1 Characteristics of pain with anatomical location

closure glaucoma. The examination should be used to rule out other causes of symptoms and should include a systemic examination.

Examination
On examination of the patient the findings include:
- the patient is sweaty and pale
- she has normal heart sounds and a regular pulse of 50 b.p.m.
- she has a soft and non-tender abdomen

The patient's pupil is shown in **Figure 12.2**.

Ophthalmic examination: The ophthalmic examination is summarised in **Table 12.2**.

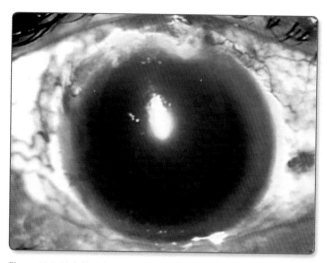

Figure 12.2 Mid-dilated pupil and corneal oedema in a patient who presented with eye pain.

Right eye		Left eye
6/6	**Visual acuity**	6/60
Normal direct, no consensual reflex	**Pupil**	Fixed and mid-dilated
Clear	**Cornea**	Hazy, difficult to see the iris features
Clear	**Anterior chamber**	Clear
Cataract	**Lens**	Cataract
Clear	**Vitreous**	Unable to see
Clear view of fundus	**Fundus**	No clear view of fundus
Normal vessels and disc	**Disc**	No view of fundus

Table 12.2 Ophthalmic examination: results for a patient who presented with eye pain

Diagnostic approach

The diagnosis of acute angle closure glaucoma is most likely from the fixed mid-dilated pupil, and this can be confirmed by an intraocular pressure check. The high intraocular pressure has probably result ed in the corneal clouding. The slow pulse, sweating and abdominal symptoms are due to activation of the vagus nerve secondary to the **oculovagal response**, a parasympathetic stimulating response when the eye is irritated.

Loss of peripheral vision

Presentation

A 70-year-old man presents to the ophthalmic outpatients department because he has been bumping into things in the periphery of his vision.

Diagnostic approach

Bilateral reduction of peripheral vision is caused by diseases affecting both retinas or optic nerves or a single lesion affecting the visual pathway beyond the optic chiasm. The history can help to characterise the nature of the peripheral visual loss, associated symptoms and risks. Although the history can point towards the differential diagnoses, the examination is key to finally reaching a diagnosis. It is important at this point to confirm whether the patient is known to already have a blind eye. If this is the case, covering the good eye may result in loss of vision.

Table 12.3 lists the clues to the diagnosis from the history.

Further history

The patient believes that the reduction in vision has been gradual and has noticed that he has been walking into things. The reduction in vision seems to affect both eyes and is in all areas of both eyes. There is no major problem with night vision.

Previous medical history: The patient has no major cardiovascular risk factors.

	Nature of field loss	Associated clues in history
Retina	Retinitis pigmentosa: peripheral constriction of the visual field	Difficulty with night vision. Possible family history
Optic nerve	Glaucoma: various patterns, including nasal field of vision, central, paracentral and peripheral alone	Family history, myopia, migraines or peripheral vasospasm, cardiovascular history
Intracerebral	Bitemporal, homonymous hemi- or quadrantinopia	Possible neurological deficit. Cerebrovascular risk factors

Table 12.3 Diagnostic clues from the history (Clinical scenario 2)

Previous ocular history: The patient has a family history of his mother having primary open angle glaucoma, but has no other ocular history other than he wears reading glasses.

Social history: The patient is a non-smoker.

Diagnostic approach

The history points towards primary open angle glaucoma. This can be confirmed with findings on examination, which should reveal a cupped optic disc. The examination should also be used to perform field tests and to examine the retina, ideally with a dilated fundus examination.

Examination

The patient has no focal neurological deficit.

Ophthalmic examination: The patient's ophthalmic examination is summarised in **Table 12.4**. **Figure 12.3** shows the patient's optic disc.

Diagnostic approach

The examination seems to exclude other causes of peripheral vision loss and points towards bilateral optic nerve pathology.

	Right eye		Left eye
	6/6	**Visual acuity**	6/6
	Peripheral visual field loss greater in the nasal area close to the central visual field	**Confrontation visual field**	Peripheral visual field loss greater in the nasal area close to the central visual field
	Normal direct and consensual reflex	**Pupil**	Normal direct and consensual reflex
	Clear	**Cornea**	Clear
	Clear	**Anterior chamber**	Clear
	Clear	**Lens**	Clear
	Clear	**Vitreous**	Clear
	Clear view of fundus No obvious retinal pathology	**Fundus**	Clear view of fundus No obvious retinal pathology
	Cupped disc with a cup to disc ratio of 0.8 No marked pallor	**Disc**	Cupped disc with a cup to disc ratio of 0.8 No marked pallor

Table 12.4 Ophthalmic examination: results for a patient who presented with loss of peripheral vision

There are various different types of optic nerve pathologies leading to a cupped disc, the most common of these being the glaucomas. Slit lamp microscopy, examination of the drainage angle, formal visual field examination and measurement of the intraocular pressure are required to confirm the diagnosis.

Sudden and complete loss of vision
Presentation
A 70-year-old woman presents to the emergency department with sudden-onset complete loss of vision in her right eye.

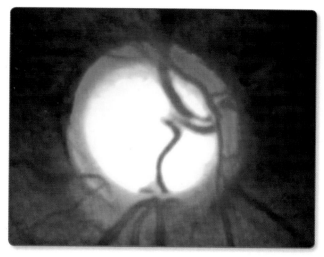

Figure 12.3 Disc cupping in a patient who presented with loss of peripheral vision.

Diagnostic approach

There are many possible causes for sudden, complete, unilateral loss of vision. Although patients complain of completeness and unilaterality, this has to be confirmed at the examination; for example, patients may have reduced vision but not complete vision loss, such as with dense cataract, or patients may not have unilateral vision loss, such as with incomplete field defects in the other eye. However, a brief, directed history can provide a number of clues to the diagnosis. This should be followed by a stepwise examination. It may then be useful to return to a more specific history, e.g. asking about vascular risk factors after discovering a central retinal artery occlusion.

Unilateral vision loss immediately excludes disease behind and including the optic chiasm. Age must be taken into consideration as certain conditions, such as optic neuritis, are far less likely in older patients (optic neuritis is generally found in those aged 20–50), but others, especially vascular disorders such as central retinal artery/vein occlusion and optic neuropathy, are far more common in older patients.

The signs and associated symptoms can help to further differentiate other diseases.

Further history

The patient states that the loss of vision was sudden, taking only minutes. There was no history of trauma and she was just watching television when she felt the vision in her right eye disappear. She has felt more tired than usual over the last couple of months and has had a long-standing headache over her right temple, but denies jaw claudication or major joint ache.

Previous medical history: The patient has hypertension and hypercholesterolaemia, and she had a myocardial infarction 3 years ago. She does not have diabetes.

Previous ocular history: The patient wears glasses for reading only.

Medications: The patient takes aspirin because of the previous myocardial infarction, bendroflumethiazide for the hypertension, and simvastatin for hypercholesterolaemia.

Diagnostic approach

Diagnosis at this stage is still not easy. The patient seems to have narrowed the time to an acute loss of vision. However, she also seems to have a history that could cover a range of different conditions, including central retinal artery occlusion, ischaemic optic neuropathy secondary to temporal arteritis, and ischaemic optic neuropathy unrelated to temporal arteritis. Of these, the most sinister is ischaemic optic neuropathy secondary to temporal arteritis.

Examination

On examination of the patient the findings include:
- temperature of 37.8°C
- heart rate of 90 b.p.m, with blood pressure 160/90 mmHg
- tenderness of the forehead, with a loss of temporal artery pulsation.

Ophthalmic examination: The patient's ophthalmic examination is summarised in **Table 12.5**. Fundoscopy shows a swollen optic disc (**Figure 12.4**).

Diagnostic approach

In this case, central retinal artery occlusion has been excluded as the blood supply appears to be unaffected. The main remaining differential diagnoses are non-arteritic ischaemic optic neuropathy and arteritic ischaemic optic neuropathy.

The diagnosis points to temporal arteritis because of the patient's age, headache, fatigue symptoms and temporal artery tenderness. Blood tests revealing a raised erythrocyte sedimentation rate (ESR), raised C-reactive protein (CRP) level and raised platelet count, which also support the diagnosis. If there is uncertainty, it is best to commence treatment with

Right eye		Left eye
No perception of light	**Visual acuity**	6/6
No response to direct and no consensual reflex Relative afferent pupillary defect Equal-sized pupils	**Pupil**	Normal direct and consensual reflex Equal-sized pupils
Clear	**Cornea**	Clear
Clear	**Anterior chamber**	Clear
Clear	**Lens**	Clear
Clear	**Vitreous**	Clear
Clear view of fundus	**Fundus**	Clear view of fundus
Disc swollen Retina normal away from disc, vessels normal	**Disc**	Normal vessels and disc

Table 12.5 Ophthalmic examination: results for a patient who presented with sudden and complete loss of vision

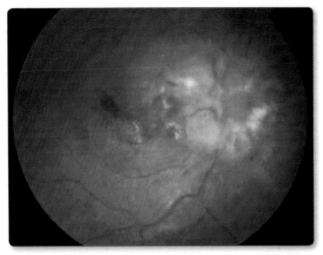

Figure 12.4 Swollen optic disc in giant cell (temporal) arteritis in a patient who presented with sudden and complete loss of vision.

high-dose corticosteroids and to arrange a biopsy of the temporal artery (see Section 12.7).

12.2 Acute angle closure glaucoma

Acute angle closure glaucoma is an ophthalmic emergency. The condition results from the mechanical closure of the aqueous drainage angle, which differentiates it from primary open angle glaucoma, a more chronic condition, in which the drainage angle is open.

Epidemiology

The risk for primary angle closure generally increases with age, peaking in the fifth and sixth decades, and is thought to be due to an increase in the size of the lens with time. There is also a marked ethnic variation, with a far higher incidence in Chinese and Indian populations than in white and Afro-Caribbean populations. Women tend to be affected slightly more often than men.

Causes

The causes of angle closure glaucoma are shown in **Table 12.6**.

Pathogenesis

Primary angle closure glaucoma: pupillary block

Over time, fibres are laid down inside the lens, causing it to thicken. This means that it gradually pushes forwards, eventually touching the iris, which lies in front of it. Eventually, this results in resistance to the flow of fluid from the ciliary body forward through the pupil. When the resistance to flow is so great that fluid cannot pass through the pupil, a phenomenon known as pupil block occurs and causes fluid to bow the iris forward occluding the **trabecular meshwork**, a sieve-like structure in the angle between the cornea and the iris (**Figure 12.5**).

Glaucoma, optic nerve damage with corresponding visual field defects, occurs as the high pressure is thought to affect blood supply to the optic nerve.

Primary angle closure glaucoma: other causes

Plateau iris is another primary cause of angle closure glaucoma. It results from an anatomical variation with anterior positioning of the root of the iris. This means that it is more likely to cause blockage of the drainage angle. As this is independent of lens size, the condition is seen in younger patients.

Secondary causes mainly result from mechanical obstruction. For example, **phacomorphic glaucoma** results

Primary angle closure	Secondary angle closure glaucoma
Pupillary block	Phacomorphic (lens expansion from a mature cataract)
Plateau iris configuration	Ciliochoroidal expansion
	Lens subluxation
	Uveitis
	Rubeiotic glaucoma

Table 12.6 Causes of angle closure glaucoma

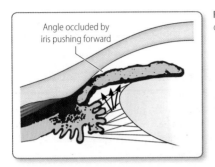

Figure 12.5 Angle closure.

Angle occluded by iris pushing forward

from bulging of a large lens, peripherally blocking outflow. Lens dislocation can cause pupil block as the mobile lens bulges forward.

Other conditions and drugs such as topiramate, an antiepileptic, are known to cause the swelling of the ciliary body and result in glaucoma by a similar mechanism.

Clinical features

Patients with acute angle closure glaucoma have a painful red eye with reduced vision and haloes around lights. Vision is reduced as the cornea becomes cloudy from being unable to pump water out into the anterior chamber. Nausea and vomiting result from activation of the vagal response.

On examination, visual acuity is reduced and the conjunctiva is red with a cloudy cornea. Pupils are fixed and mid-dilated and often it is not possible to view the fundus (**Figure 12.6**). Examination of the angle with a gonioscope lens will reveal a closed angle. Intraocular pressure is high, usually varying from 40 to 70 mmHg.

Examination should also include a risk assessment of the other eye.

Risk factors

The risk factors for acute angle closure glaucoma include:

> ## Clinical insight
>
> Activation of the oculovagal response causes an increased systemic parasympathetic response. It is not uncommon to see patients with a low pulse who are sweaty, pale and vomiting and complaining of abdominal pain.

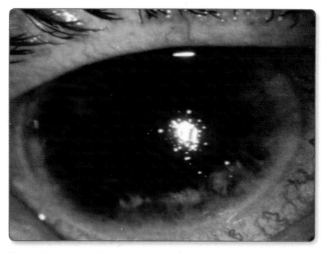

Figure 12.6 An eye with angle closure and fixed mid-dilated pupil with an oedematous cornea.

- a shallow anterior chamber
- hypermetropia
- a short eye
- older age
- the presence of cataract
- a small cornea
- anticholinergics, e.g. tricyclic antidepressants

Differential diagnosis

Once high intraocular pressure is established in a painful eye with a reduction in vision, the main differential diagnoses are between different types of acute glaucomas:

- *plateau iris*: usually occurs in younger patients, and recurs despite iridotomy
- *phacomorphic glaucoma*: dense cataract is present
- *inflammatory glaucoma*: there are posterior synechiae around the pupil margin, with cellular activity in the anterior chamber; in addition, the iris bows forward (known as iris bombé)

- *neovascular glaucoma*: there is other retinal pathology, e.g. diabetes or retinal vein occlusion, or new vessels on the iris and in the drainage angle

Management

The aim of medical management initially is to reduce intraocular pressure. A combination of topical drops and intravenous medications such as acetazolamide and mannitol are used to lower intraocular pressure. Pilocarpine, a parasympathomimetic, is added topically to reduce the size of the pupil.

Once normal pressure is achieved and the cornea clears, a laser **iridotomy** (i.e. a hole in the iris) can be performed as definitive management. This enables aqueous to flow from the ciliary body through the iris to the trabecular meshwork, consequently bypassing any pupil block. Very rarely, if the cornea does not clear, a surgical **peripheral iridectomy** is performed for the same effect, where a part of the iris is removed.

Prognosis

The visual prognosis is usually good if the symptoms and signs are spotted early and treatment instigated. However, any delay in the diagnosis and prolonged high intraocular pressure result in permanent visual field defects. Annual follow-up is the norm in order to document visual fields and to ensure patency of peripheral iridotomies.

12.3 Chronic open angle glaucoma

This section discusses open angle glaucoma, normal tension glaucoma and ocular hypertension.

Open angle glaucoma encompasses a range of common, potentially blinding diseases. These diseases are defined by the observation of optic neuropathy and glaucomatous field defects in the presence of an open aqueous drainage angle. However, intraocular pressure does not necessarily have to be raised for glaucoma to be diagnosed, e.g. **normal tension glaucoma**. Unlike angle closure glaucoma, field defects usually develop slowly and therefore long-term monitoring is key. Raised intraocular pressure without any field defects or observable disc changes is called **ocular hypertension**.

Epidemiology

Approximately 10% of people over the age of 75 have primary open angle glaucoma, constituting 10% of blind registrations. Normal tension glaucoma constitutes approximately one quarter of these cases. Although there is no sex association, the disease is more prevalent among those of Afro-Caribbean descent.

In the population over the age of 40, 5–10% are thought to have ocular hypertension.

Pathogenesis

The exact mechanism of glaucoma is unknown. However, several theories have developed from the finding that modifying intraocular pressure alters the risk of glaucoma. The major hypothesis is that higher intraocular pressure reduces blood flow to the optic nerve head, which results in subsequent nerve loss. This may also explain why some patients with cardiovascular risk factors and hence vessel disease have glaucoma despite normal intraocular pressures.

Raised intraocular pressure is thought to result from increasing resistance to the flow of aqueous in the trabecular meshwork with time.

Clinical features

Open angle glaucoma is asymptomatic until its late stages and loss of vision is irreversible. Patients may describe loss of peripheral vision, resulting in them bumping into things. Others may lose central vision.

Because of the incipient nature of onset, regular visits to an optometrist are important in order to screen for the condition, especially in those with risk factors. When questioning patients, it is important ask about risk factors, not only for the risk of glaucoma but also for the risk of progression.

Examination includes:
- an intraocular pressure check,
- optic nerve visualisation
- visual field testing

Examination usually reveals a white, normal-looking eye with a clear cornea. Examination of the drainage angle with a **gonioscope**, a special contact lens that allows viewing of the drainage angle, is unremarkable.

Patients suspected of having glaucoma should be referred to hospital eye services for a full examination.

Intraocular pressure
Intraocular pressure can be checked most accurately with a **Goldman tonometer**, a spring-loaded pressure-measuring device. In new patients, the thickness of the cornea should be measured (**pachymetry**), as variations in thickness alter the measured intraocular pressure and may give a false reading.

Optic nerve visualisation
The optic disc is usually cupped (**Figure 12.7**).

Visual field testing
Visual field testing should be performed. **Figure 12.8** shows a common visual field defect in early glaucoma. Recent developments in **ocular coherence tomography**, an ophthalmic scanning method using infrared light rays, mean that the retinal nerve layers can be easily visualised and monitored. This may give additional information about progression.

Diagnostic criteria
Open angle glaucoma encompasses a spectrum of disease, the boundaries of which are listed in **Table 12.7**. In reality, there is often blurring of the boundaries, e.g. when diagnosing whether a disc is cupped or not.

Risk factors
The risk factors for chronic open angle glaucoma include:
- high intraocular pressure
- older age
- Afro-Caribbean ancestry
- family history of glaucoma
- myopia

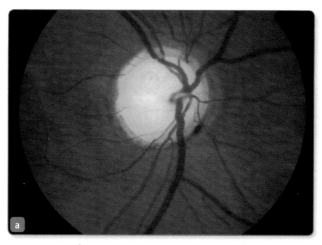

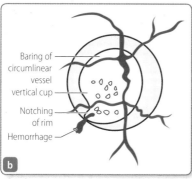

Baring of
circumlinear
vessel
vertical cup
Notching
of rim
Hemorrhage

Figure 12.7a A glaucomatous cupped disc. (Courtesy of the medical photography department, Princess Alexandra Eye Pavilion, Edinburgh).

- peripheral vasospasm
- migraine
- systemic hypertension
- cardiovascular disease
- diabetes

Differential diagnosis

The initial differential diagnoses define the type of glaucoma/ocular hypertension disease:

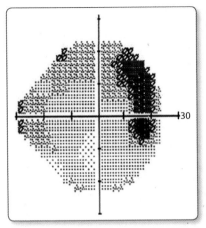

Figure 12.8 A common early visual field defect in glaucoma, as indicated by the shaded areas.

	Ocular hypertension	Primary open angle glaucoma	Normal tension glaucoma
Intraocular pressure	>21	>21	<21
Optic nerve	Normal	Cupping	Cupping
Visual field	Normal	Defects	Defects

Table 12.7 Diagnostic criteria for open angle glaucoma and ocular hypertension

- *secondary glaucomas*: there is pigment on the cornea, deposits on the lens and iris transillumination (see Section 12.4)
- *compressive optic neuropathy*: atypical field defect, pallor greater than cupping and greatly asymmetrical field loss
- *optic neuropathies*: look for systemic diseases, such as systemic lupus erythematosus (SLE), syphilis, sarcoidosis, or vitamin B_1, B_2, B_6 and B_{12} deficiencies. Many of these diseases can be screened for by relevant blood tests if suspected and the diagnosis of glaucoma is not clear

Management

Intraocular pressure is the main modifiable glaucoma risk factor. Consequently, treatment centres on lowering intraocular pressure.

Medical

There are now a wide variety of drops available to either decrease aqueous production or increase the outflow of aqueous from the eye. Decisions about drops should take account of their side-effect profile.

Laser

Laser procedures can be used in patients who cannot tolerate drops. They have been shown to control intraocular pressure in over two thirds of patients initially, although success reduces with time. The mechanism of action is incompletely understood, although it is thought that it directly increases aqueous outflow via the trabecular meshwork.

Surgery

When other interventions fail, surgery is attempted. The most common glaucoma operation is the **trabeculectomy**. This is when a trapdoor-like incision is made into the sclera under the conjunctiva (**Figure 12.9**). When intraocular pressure increases, the trapdoor flap opens, allowing fluid to drain out under the conjunctiva.

When trabeculectomy is repeatedly unsuccessful, an intraocular tube with an externally linked valve can be used to control intraocular pressure.

Prognosis

The prognosis for open angle glaucoma is good if disease is diagnosed early and there is good treatment compliance. The 5-year untreated conversion rate of ocular hypertension to glaucoma is approximately 10%. In normal tension glaucoma, almost half of the patients do not progress even if left untreated.

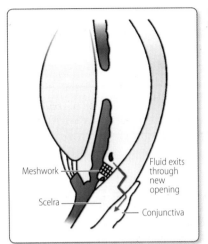

Figure 12.9 The trabeculectomy procedure.

Meshwork

Scelra

Fluid exits through new opening

Conjunctiva

12.4 Secondary glaucomas

Secondary glaucomas cover a range of differing conditions that are linked by a primary disease resulting in secondary raised intraocular pressure (**Table 12.8**), with resultant optic neuropathy and glaucomatous visual field loss. Examples include:

- corticosteroid-induced glaucoma
- pigmentary glaucoma in pigment dispersion syndrome (**Figure 12.10**)
- protein deposition in pseudoexfoliation syndrome (**Figure 12.11**)
- ischaemic eye disease resulting in iris new vessels (**Figure 12.12**)

For treatment of uveitic glaucoma, see Chapter 10.

12.5 Optic neuritis

Optic neuritis is an acute demyelinating disease of the optic nerve. It is the most common cause of unilateral painful vision loss in a young adult.

	Pigment dispersion syndrome	Pseudoexfoliation	Rubeiotic glaucoma	Corticosteroid-induced glaucoma
Epidemiology	Onset of glaucoma is usually in the third or fourth decade. More common in young men	Found in approximately 10% of the general population. Glaucoma usually presents after the age of 40	Found in 1% of patients with diabetes	Approximately one third of patients on long-term steroid drops
Aetiology	Dominantly inherited disease	Polygenic and complex disease Systemic condition resulting from shedding of dandruff-like material from organs	Secondary to ischaemia of the eye from retinal vein occlusion, diabetes or a stenosed carotid artery	Increased risk in those with pre-existing glaucoma
Pathogenesis	Pigment released as lens zonules rub against the iris. Released pigment blocks the outflow of aqueous	Shed material is deposited in the drainage angle, reducing aqueous outflow	Release of blood vessel growth factors from ischaemic tissue results in new blood vessels that eventually grow and fibrose in the drainage angle, preventing aqueous outflow	Unknown mechanism. Thought to lead to structural changes that cause increased resistance to outflow in the trabecular meshwork
Clinical features	Patients are usually asymptomatic. However, some may complain of ache after exercise and acute pigment release. Examination	Patients are usually asymptomatic. Examination reveals transillumination around the edge of the pupil. Dilation is poor and there is	Patients complain of blurring and pain. Iris shows new vessels (see **Figure 12.12**). There are vessels in the angle on gonioscopy. Usually,	Known recent use of topical or oral corticosteroid. Examination reveals no other obvious abnormalities

	with a gonioscope reveals pigment on the cornea and in the angle. Mid-peripheral iris transillumination (see **Figure 12.10**)	usually obvious deposit inside the pupil border (see **Figure 12.11**). Gonioscopy reveals pigment deposition in the trabeculum	there is retinal pathology in the form of haemorrhages or new vessels	
Management	Topical treatment to reduce intraocular pressure if raised. Laser treatment to the trabecular meshwork works well in most initially. If this fails, a trabeculectomy is attempted	Similar to pigment dispersion syndrome	Early treatment of the ischaemic tissue with laser photocoagulation to try to reverse new vessel formation. Carotid endarterectomy for carotid disease. Increasingly, intraocular injection of antibodies to vascular growth factors are used to try to reduce new vessel formation. Topical treatment is used to control intraocular pressure	Reduce or stop corticosteroid. Otherwise, treat as primary open angle glaucoma
Prognosis	Approximately one third of patients develop glaucoma	Approximately one quarter of patients develop glaucoma	Poor prognosis owing to uncontrollable pressure, poor vision and pain	Good if identified early

Table 12.8 Comparison of types of secondary glaucoma

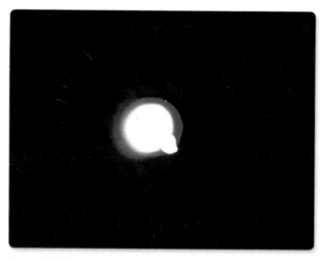

Figure 12.10 Transillumination in pigment dispersion syndrome.

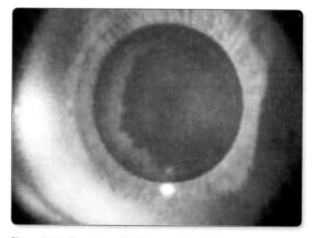

Figure 12.11 Deposition of fibrillar material on the lens in pseudoexfoliation.

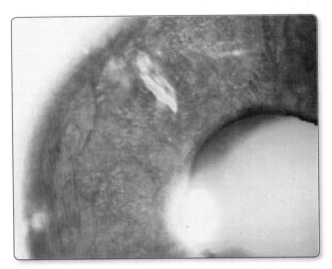

Figure 12.12 New vessels on the iris in rubeiotic glaucoma.

Epidemiology

The approximate incidence of optic neuritis is 5 per 100,000 per year with a prevalence of 115 per 100,000 in the UK; these figures are similar to those for multiple sclerosis (MS). Optic neuritis is three times as common in females as in males, with patients generally ranging between 20 and 45 years old. Like MS it is more commonly seen in caucasian populations.

Causes

Optic neuritis is closely linked to MS, although in the young it may be secondary to viral illness.

Pathogenesis

Optic neuritis is thought to result from localised inflammation caused by delayed type hypersensitivity. Lymphocytes cross the blood–brain barrier and inflammation results in the loss of myelin. Demyelination results in the reduction and delay of optic nerve conduction.

Clinical features

The clinical features of optic neuritis include:

- loss of vision for usually 7–10 days, varying from mild reduction to loss of light perception
- periocular pain, which is classically retrobulbar (90%) and is exacerbated by movement
- loss of colour vision
- visual field loss with various field defects, including altitudinal, arcuate and nasal field loss

Fundoscopy reveals nerve swelling (**Figure 12.13**) in one third of cases with the other two thirds being retrobulbar.

In children, optic neuritis can occur during or after viral infection and is bilateral in 70% of cases.

Diagnostic criteria

The diagnostic criteria for optic neuritis as per the Optic Neuritis Treatment Trial include:

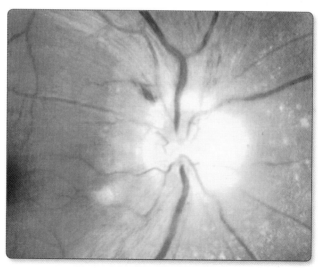

Figure 12.13 Optic nerve swelling in optic neuritis.

- the typical symptoms of optic neuritis, as found in the Optic Neuritis Treatment Trial

> ### Clinical insight
> Loss of colour vision is often out of proportion to loss of vision initially.

- an acute onset, with progression over a few days
- unilateral occurrence (70%)
- reduced contrast and colour vision
- periocular pain (90%)
- patients are usually aged 20–45
- a relative afferent pupillary defect (RAPD)
- spontaneous improvement in >90% of patients in 2 weeks

Investigations

Further investigation of a first case of typical optic neuritis is not always warranted. However, if there are features of atypical optic neuritis or of a differential diagnosis, it is important to carry out a full assessment with referral to the neuro-ophthalmology department.

Initial investigations include blood tests to rule out common differential diagnoses. There should also be radiological investigations, including MRI. This will assist in excluding some differential diagnoses, such as compressive optic neuropathy, in cases of atypical optic neuritis.

Lumbar puncture is usually reserved for children and for bilateral and atypical cases.

Differential diagnosis

The differential diagnoses for optic neuritis include:

- *compressive optic neuropathy*: there is a slow onset and early pallor to the disc
- *inflammatory optic neuropathies, e.g. sarcoidosis, SLE*: there are systemic signs of disease, with raised inflammatory and connective tissue markers
- *anterior ischaemic optic neuropathy*: the colour vision is usually less affected, there is an altitudinal field defect, and only half of the disc is swollen

- *toxic causes, e.g. vitamin B$_{12}$ deficiency*: there is pallor to the disc, which is reversible with high-dose vitamin supplementation
- *inherited causes, e.g. Leber hereditary optic neuropathy*: there is sudden onset, with sequential changes

Management

Although high-dose intravenous corticosteroids do improve short-term recovery of vision they do not provide benefit in the long term with regard to progression or recurrence. Thus, treatment should be undertaken after a discussion with the patient about preferences versus the risk of side-effects. At present, there is no significant evidence for the use of intravenous immunoglobulins, unlike in MS.

Prognosis

Usually, vision begins to improve by 3 weeks in 80% of patients, and continues to improve for up to 1 year. At 1 year vision is 6/12 or better in the affected eye in 90% of patiets The visual prognosis is better in those who initially lose the least vision. Patients will, however, continue to have colour and contrast difficulties. Patients commonly ask about the risk of MS; this increases with optic neuritis and with the number of periventricular white matter lesions found on brain MRI (**Table 12.9**).

12.6 Optic atrophy

Optic atrophy describes the final phenotype of many diseases that result in loss of neurones from the geniculate nucleus

Optic neuritis	MRI brain	Risk (15 years)
Yes	No lesions	25%
Yes	1 lesion	60%
Yes	2 lesions	68%
Yes	>2 lesions	78%

Table 12.9 Risk of developing multiple sclerosis (data from Optic Neuritis Study Group. Arch Neurol 2008;65:727–32).

to the ganglion cells in the retina. The loss of these neurones also leads to loss of retrograde cells in the retina, and hence also brings about the visual changes associated with atrophy.

Epidemiology
The prevalence of optic atrophy is about 0.1% in the older population. Optic atrophy is slightly more prevalent among the Afro-Caribbean population.

Causes
The causes of optic atrophy are listed in **Table 12.10**.

Pathogenesis
The optic nerve cells originate at the ganglion cells and course to the lateral geniculate nucleus. Since they are non-regenerative, damage gradually reduces their number, eventually leading to optic atrophy. Therefore, this is not the pathological definition of atrophy but more a degeneration. The pallor seen in the optic nerve is thought to come from the altered reflectance

Intrinsic/extrinsic	Type of disease	Examples of disease
Intrinsic	Nutritional/toxic	B_1, B_2, B_6, B_{12} and folate deficiency Methanol, ethambutol, amiodarone and toxicity
	Inflammatory	SLE, sarcoidosis, temporal arteritis
	Vascular	Central retinal artery occlusion
	Infective	Syphilis, TB
	Inherited	Leber hereditary optic neuropathy
Extrinsic	Compression	Tumour Glaucoma
	Traumatic	Axonal damage from external head trauma

SLE, systemic lupus erythematosus; TB, tuberculosis.

Table 12.10 Causes of optic atrophy

of degenerated neurones and the reduction in the number of small blood vessels at the optic nerve head.

Clinical features

Patients may describe various rates of painless reduction in vision depending on disease origin. Generally, vascular diseases and diseases such as Leber's hereditary optic atrophy have a fairly rapid onset, whereas nutritional or toxic causes result in an insidious onset. A family history is important in inherited conditions.

Examination reveals reduced central vision and colour vision. Well-performed confrontation visual field testing may help to identify the initial central visual field loss. Fundoscopy shows a pale and cupped disc (**Figure 12.14**). The intraocular pressure should be measured to determine whether the cause is glaucomatous.

Investigations

Investigations should concentrate on the diagnosis, especially of reversible causes. Initially, this can include simple blood tests for vitamin deficiencies, an inflammatory and connective

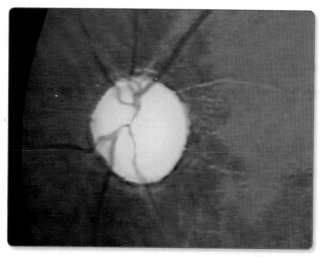

Figure 12.14 Optic atrophy.

tissue screen and blood tests for infective causes. Unilateral asymmetrical atrophy should prompt MRI or CT scanning of the orbit and head.

Differential diagnosis

The differential diagnoses include other causes of pale disc:
- *myelinated nerve fibres in the retina*: this usually goes beyond the area of the disc in one segment
- *coloboma*: this may be associated with inferior retinal and pupillary changes
- *optic disc pit*: there is a pale disc with greyish-coloured pit
- *optic disc drusen*: there is a raised yellowish disc

Management

Nutritional disorders can be treated with high-dose vitamin supplementation. Inflammatory disorders may require high-dose corticosteroid treatment to protect the other eye. Finally, surgery may be indicated for external compressive tumours.

Prognosis

The condition is currently untreatable and irreversible, and thus has a poor prognosis

12.7 Anterior ischaemic optic neuropathy

Anterior ischaemic optic neuropathy (AION) is an occlusive condition of the blood supply to the anterior optic nerve and optic nerve head. The condition is divided by cause into **arteritic** (secondary to arteritis, most commonly giant cell (temporal) arteritis) and **non-arteritic** (i.e. not caused by inflammation to the blood vessel). These are two different diseases affecting similar anatomical areas. The arteritic type is an ophthalmic emergency because of the high risk of complete loss of vision if left untreated.

Epidemiology

AION secondary to temporal arteritis affects individuals over the age of 50. The incidence is approximately 10 per 100,000 per year in this age group. Of cases occur in Caucasian populations. It is twice as common in women. Only 10% of AION is caused by artertic types, the rest resulting from non-arteritic causes.

Causes

Arteritic AION is usually caused by temporal arteritis. Rarely, other causes of **vasculitis**, i.e. inflammation of the blood vessels such as in polyarteritis nodosa and Churg–Strauss syndrome (allergic granulomatosis), have been reported.

Pathogenesis

Temporal arteritis is an inflammatory disease of unknown aetiology affecting small- to medium-sized arteries. These include the vessels of the forehead (superficial temporal arteries) and ocular blood vessels (short posterior ciliary, ophthalmic, central retinal and choroidal arteries). Inflammation leads to thickening of arterial walls, ultimately leading to occlusion, ischaemia and necrosis of downstream tissue (**Figure 12.15**).

The pathogenesis of non-arteritic disease is unclear. Various proposals have included microembolism, arteriosclerosis and vasospasm. However, like arteritic disease, the final outcome is the loss of blood flow to the optic nerve head.

Clinical features

Arteritic AION

The prodromal features of arteritic AION include:

- headache (in 50% of cases)
- scalp tenderness
- weight loss
- fatigue
- anorexia
- low-grade fever
- jaw claudication and neck pain

Arteritic AION presents with rapid, severe loss of vision, usually resulting in a RAPD. About one quarter of patients

Guiding principle

Patients may complain of a number of vague symptoms prior to arteritic anterior ischaemic optic neuropathy (AION). It is important to have a low threshold of suspicion when these symptoms are mentioned as arteritic AION is an ophthalmological emergency and can cause blindness.

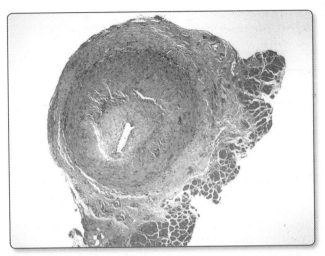

Figure 12.15 Cross-section of an artery in temporal arteritis. Courtesy of Dr Coline Smith, Neuropathology Unit, Western General Hospital, Edinburgh.

have transient vision loss prior to AION. Eventual vision loss is poorer than 6/60 in 75% of patients. In the acute stages, the optic disc is usually pale and swollen (**Figure 12.16**).

Clinical insight

It is important to note that polymyalgia rheumatica, an inflammatory disease of the girdle muscles, increases the risk of temporal arteritis.

Non-arteritic AION

Non-arteritic AION usually has no preceding symptoms and presents with sudden painless blurring of vision; however, 10% of patients do have an ache around the eye after the event. Vision is less severely affected than in arteritic AION, with 60% of patients having vision better than 6/60. In the majority of cases, there is a RAPD with swelling of the optic nerve, often accompanied by haemorrhages around the disc.

The majority of patients have an altitudinal field loss, in which only the top or bottom half of the visual field is reduced.

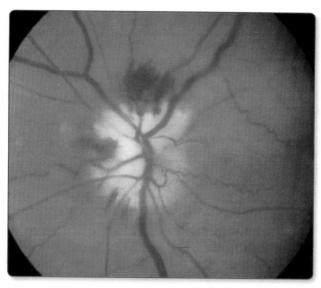

Figure 12.16 The disc in anterior ischaemic optic neuropathy.

Diagnostic criteria

The British Society for Rheumatology describes key features that enable clinical diagnosis:

· an abrupt new headache
· scalp pain and tenderness
· jaw claudication
· visual symptoms, e.g. diplopia
· symptoms of polymyalgia rheumatica
· temporal artery abnormalities
· raised ESR and CRP level

Risk factors

The risk factors for non-arteritic AION include:

· hypertension
· diabetes
· ischaemic heart disease

· hypercholesterolaemia
· a crowded (non-cupped) optic disc

Investigations

If the ESR, CRP level and platelet count are raised, there is an increased risk of temporal arteritis (**Table 12.11**). However, if there is still diagnostic uncertainty, patients are usually given treatment while awaiting a temporal artery biopsy, which remains the gold standard. There is no reason to delay treatment as biopsy signs of temporal arteritis can still be noted up to 2 weeks after commencement of steroid treatment.

In non-arteritic AION, the cardiovascular risk factors should be assessed in order to prevent recurrence of disease. Tests include blood pressure, full blood count, serum glucose and lipid screen. In those under the age of 50, a coagulation and vasculitis screen may be considered. Visual field testing can help to diagnose and monitor vision.

Differential diagnosis

The features of arteritic and non-arteritic AION are compared in **Table 12.12** (see **Figure 3.2** for other differential diagnoses).

Management
Arteritic AION

The mainstay of management of AION is a high-dose systemic corticosteroid with the main aim of preventing loss of vision in the contralateral eye. Although oral corticosteroids (e.g. 1–1.5 mg/

Test	Sensitivity (%)	Specificity (%)
ESR	94.2	80.5
CRP level	98.6	75.7
Platelet count	57.0	96.5
CRP, C-reactive protein; ESR, erythrocyte sedimentation rate.		

Table 12.11 Sensitivity and specificity of haematological tests in temporal arteritis (data from Costello et al. Eur J Opthalmol 2004;14:245–57)

	Arteritic AION	**Non-arteritic AION**
Age	>50	50–70
Pain	Headache	Painless
Loss of vision	Sudden, severe loss	Sudden, usually less severe
Optic disc	Swollen and pale acutely Pale and cupped later	Swollen with haemorrhages Little cupping later
Visual field loss	Altitudinal/complete	Altitudinal
Recovery	Poor. Risk to contralateral eye	Almost half have some visual improvement
Blood tests	Raised ESR, CRP level and platelet count	Normal
Prognosis	Poor unless treated early	Up to 40% improve spontaneously
CRP, C-reactive protein; ESR, erythrocyte sedimentation rate.		

Table 12.12 Comparison of arteritic and non-arteritic anterior ischaemic optic neuropathy (AION)

kg prednisolone) have been used acutely, there is an increasing trend towards using intravenous therapy for the first 3 days (e.g. 1 g methylprednisolone) before reverting to oral maintenance. Symptoms usually resolve within 24 h.

Regular review with further ESR testing is required as there is a risk of recurrence during corticosteroid tapering. Corticosteroid is tapered slowly, usually over a year, although some patients have to be maintained on low doses indefinitely. Because of the age range of patients, it is important not to forget bone and gastric protection when prescribing corticosteroids, and dual-emission X-ray absorptiometry (DEXA) scans should be carried out to check for osteoporosis according to local policy.

Non-arteritic AION

There is no proven treatment for non-arteritic AION. However, aspirin is often prescribed to reduce the risk in the other eye.

Prognosis

The visual prognosis in arteritic AION is very poor unless treatment is delivered swiftly. In contrast, non-arteritic AION has a far better prognosis: initial vision is better and approximately 40% of patients notice an improvement in vision of up to three Snellen chart lines after 6 months.

12.8 Papilloedema

Papilloedema describes a swollen optic nerve head secondary to raised intracranial pressure.

Epidemiology

Papilloedema is a rare condition with no obvious race or sex predilection.

Causes

The causes of papilloedema (some of which are shown in **Table 12.13**) are closely linked to the causes of raised intracranial pressure.

Types of raised intracranial pressure	Causes
Mass effect	Tumour Haemorrhage Abscess
Generalised brain swelling	Idiopathic intracranial hypertension Liver failure Reye syndrome Malignant hypertension
Increased CSF production	Meningitis
Reduced CSF outflow	Arnold–Chiari malformation (cerebellomedullary malformation syndrome) Aqueductal stenosis
Increased venous pressure	Sinus thrombosis
CSF, cerebrospinal fluid.	

Table 12.13 Causes of papilloedema

Pathogenesis

Papilloedema describes swelling of the optic nerve head. The optic nerve is surrounded by a sheath. Between the nerve fibres and the sheath runs cerebrospinal fluid, which is continuous with the subarachnoid space. Thus, raised intracranial pressure compresses the nerve, causing optic nerve head oedema and accumulation of returning cerebrospinal fluid.

Clinical features

Patients initially may be asymptomatic. If there are systemic symptoms, these usually include headache and nausea, which are classically worse on lying down. In addition, there may be pulsatile tinnitus. Ocular symptoms include transient bilateral obscurations of vision several times a day and, later, reduced vision. Examination reveals reduced vision later in disease, and confrontation visual field testing may reveal an enlarged blind spot. Fundoscopy shows swollen optic discs (**Figure 12.17**).

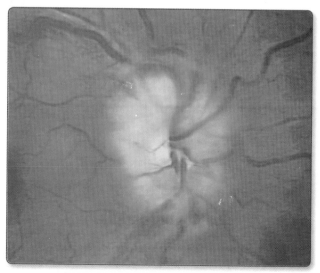

Figure 12.17 Established disc papilloedema.

Investigations

The investigations for papilloedema include:
- urgent CT with contrast or MRI with gadolinium
- MR venography to rule out cerebral sinus thrombosis
- lumbar puncture if radiology is negative

Differential diagnosis

The differential diagnoses for a swollen optic disc are listed in **Table 12.14**.

> **Guiding principle**
>
> The most important diagnosis to exclude when papilloedema is noticed is a space-occupying lesion.

Management

Management depends on the specific cause. The most common cause is idiopathic intracranial hypertension. This can be treated initially with weight loss and withdrawal of offending medications, e.g. tetracycline and the oral contraceptive pill. If these are ineffective, high-dos e regular acetazolamide can be used to reduce cerebrospinal fluid production. If other measures are ineffective, a neurosurgical shunt procedure can be used to mechanically divert cerebrospinal fluid.

Mass lesions require specific treatment, including excision, chemotherapy or radiotherapy when indicated for tumours and drainage for haemorrhage and abscess when required.

Unilateral	Bilateral
Early optic neuritis: marked reduction in colour vision and visual acuity	Disc drusen: asymmetric; ultrasound used to diagnose
Anterior ischaemic optic neuropathy: marked reduction in visual field	Hypermetropic prescription
Tumour: CT or MRI diagnosis	
Diabetic papillitis: usually in young patients; unilateral with vision maintained and spontaneous resolution	

Table 12.14 Differential diagnoses of disc swelling

Prognosis

Loss of vision from papilloedema is rare if management is initiated promptly. A recent UK survey found an incidence of only 2% of those with legal blindness in cases of idiopathic intracranial hypertension.

12.9 Visual pathway defects

Light perception occurs when light is converted to an electrical signal by photoreceptors; this signal is then transmitted to bipolar and then to ganglion cells. The signal is transmitted along the optic nerve before joining the optic tract. The neurones synapse at the thalamus, resulting in optic radiations that travel to the occipital lobe for final processing. There is also a partial crossing over of visual pathways at the chiasm. Defects can occur anywhere along this pathway, leading to visual field defects. This section related to the common defects behind the optic nerve head (**Figure 12.18**).

Causes

The causes of visual pathway defects include:

- ischaemia
- haemorrhage
- compression (e.g. tumours or abscesses)
- trauma
- nutritional abnormalities (e.g. vitamin B_6 and B_{12} deficiency)
- toxicity

Pathogenesis

Defects result from disruption of nerve conduction. Partial or early loss may lead to positive phenomena such as photopsia (i.e. flashing lights). Late or complete disruption leads to complete loss of transmission, causing negative phenomena and deficits in the field of vision.

Clinical features

Patients may have loss of vision. This is especially true of defects affecting the central visual field, whereas other defects may

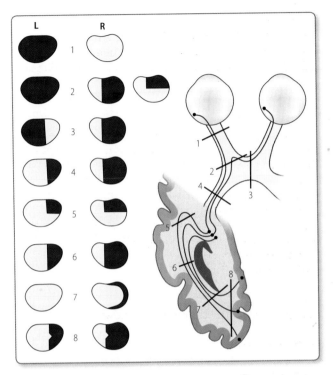

Figure 12.18 The pathways and defects in the visual field. (1) Lesion through optic nerve—ipsilateral blindness. (2) Lesion through proximal part of optic nerve—ipsilateral blindness with contralateral hemianopia. (3) Sagittal lesion of chiasma—bitemporal hemianopia. (4) Lesion of optic tract—homonymous hemianopia. (5) Lesion of temporal lobe—quadrantic homonymous defect. (6) Lesion of optic radiations—homonymous hemianopia (sometimes sparing the macula). (7) Lesion in anterior part of occipital cortex—contralateral temporal crescentic field defect. (8) Lesion of occipital lobe—homonymous hemianopia (usually sparing the macula)

go unnoticed. Examination will reveal reduced vision if central vision is affected. Confrontation visual field testing should elucidate defects and help to correlate the sites of cerebral lesions (see Section 2.2).

Clinical insight

Clues to the anatomical location of the lesion include:

· *congruency:* i.e. how similar the shape of the visual field defects are; congruency increases the more posterior the lesion is towards the occiput

· *macular sparing:* this occurs in more posterior lesions

· *homonymous defects:* in which the same side of the visual field is affected in both eyes; this occurs in defects posterior to the chiasm

Investigations

Formal visual field testing should be performed to first diagnose a defect and then to monitor progression.

Other investigations involve those for cerebral infarction and routine blood tests, including fasting cholesterol and glucose. Additionally, prompt imaging in the form of contrast-enhanced CT to diagnose the site of the lesion and to exclude space-occupying lesions.

Differential diagnosis

Atypical visual field defects may be difficult to differentiate from retinal or optic nerve pathology. The main differential diagnoses are:

· *glaucoma*: this is usually slowly progressive with disc changes

· *retinoschisis*: there are cyst-like swellings in the peripheral retina

· **optic disc drusen:** usually the optic nerve head is swollen

Management

Management varies with the underlying cause:

· infarction secondary to cardiovascular disease or embolus requires a full cardiac work-up in order to exclude sources and to determine the management of modifiable risk factors

· intracerebral space-occupying lesions require urgent neurosurgical follow-up

Disability can be reduced by teaching patients to make adjustments. For instance, in homonymous hemianopias, patients should turn their entire head towards the side of the deficit. Prisms can also be used to enhance the field of view

Prognosis

The prognosis is poor for deficits as the central nervous system does not regenerate. This has specific implications for certain occupations, including heavy goods vehicle drivers, pilots and military personnel, who have stringent visual guidelines for employment.

Ocular motility and pupils

The majority of functions required for good vision are controlled automatically. To see binocularly, both eyes need vision. In addition, both eyes need to focus at approximately the same point in space.

Sensory fusion is when the brain merges images from the two eyes even though the eyes may be aimed at slightly different points in space. However, binocular vision also requires **motor fusion**, in which the eyes mechanically point in the same direction; otherwise, sensory fusion may break down with increasing disparity of images. This is similar to the feeling one gets when one slowly crosses one's eyes.

Stereovision is a layer of information added to binocular vision to take account of depth cues. Breakdown of this system occurs commonly and can lead to double vision. If this occurs in the young, it can lead to permanent loss of vision, known as amblyopia, as the brain attempts to suppress stereovision (see Chapter 14); if it occurs in adults, it results in double vision.

Terminology of ocular motility

A **squint** is when the eyes do not point in the same direction. It is also known as **strabismus** and can be **concomitant**, in which the angle remains the same in all fields of gaze, or **incomitant**, in which the angle between the eyes varies in different positions of gaze.

A squint can be manifest, in which an angle of deviation is noted in normal gaze, or it can be latent. Manifest strabismus is associated with -**tropias** whereas latent strabismus is associated with -**phorias**, as descriptions of eye movements. These can be **exo-** (divergent angle between the eyes), **eso-** (convergent angle between the eyes), **hypo-** (one eye is lower than the other) or **hyper-** (one eye is superior to the other); for example, a manifest strabismus with a divergent angle is known as an exotropia.

Anatomy and physiology

Eye movements

Eye movements are controlled by various centres in the brain and include slow, steady pursuit or rapid, jerky, sudden bursts. In addition, the vestibular system provides input to orientate the eyes according to head position. A further centre co-ordinates convergence via the oculomotor nuclei.

To perform eye movements synchronously, feedback control from blur centres in the occipital area relay information to the motor nuclei of cranial nerves II (optic nerve), IV (trochlear nerve) and VI (abducent nerve). When moving to find a target, the innervations of the eye work as a modified pulley. The action of the activating muscle of one eye is matched by the action of the activating muscle in the contralateral eye. Equally, the inhibition of the relaxing muscle of one eye is matched by the inhibition of the relaxing muscle in the contralateral eye in order to maintain synchronous movements.

Pupil constriction and dilatation

The musculature of the pupil controls pupil size by means of the radially orientated dilator pupillae and the concentrically arranged sphincter pupillae. The amount of light entering the eye is controlled autonomically.

The pupil constricts with parasympathetic activity. Pupil constriction is part of a reflex loop whose afferent fibres travel along the outside of the optic nerve to the Edinger–Westphal nucleus (accessory parasympathetic nucleus) of the third cranial nerve (oculomotor nerve) in the midbrain, before travelling along the third cranial nerve to supply the efferent fibres to the iris sphincter muscle (**Figure 13.1**).

The pupil dilates with sympathetic stimulation. This requires uninterrupted innervation from the sympathetic centres in the midbrain via the sympathetic plexus in the neck to the iris (**Figure 13.2**).

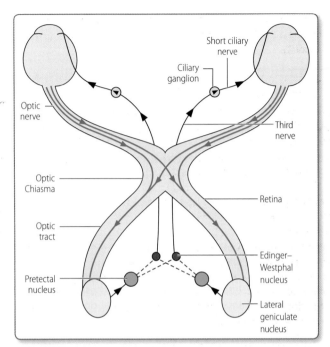

Figure 13.1 Pupillary constriction pathways.

The balance of sympathetic and parasympathetic stimulation is in constant flux at any given state of retinal illumination.

13.1 Clinical scenarios

New-onset double vision

Presentation

A 56-year-old woman presents to the emergency department with new-onset double vision.

Diagnostic approach

The aim is to determine from the history, first, whether this is true binocular double vision or whether it is monocular double vision. If it is binocular, it is useful to determine which

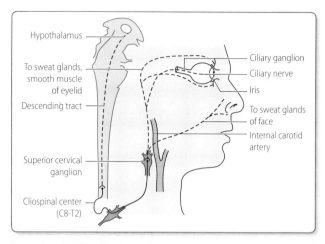

Figure 13.2 Pupillary dilatation pathways.

muscles have been affected and then to assess the possible mechanism of the weakness. In horizontal double vision, a sixth nerve palsy is most likely. Vertical double vision relates to the vertical muscles being involved. A search for other related neurology, such as hemiparesis, may also help to isolate the cause of the weakness.

In terms of the mechanism, the most common cause of new double vision at this age is microvascular damage, so a history of cardiovascular risk factors should be sought as well as any history of trauma.

Diagnostic clues in the history: With new-onset double vision in an adult, the cause is likely to be an incomitant or a paralytic squint, i.e. one in which the angle of deviation varies in different positions of gaze. In this age group, microvascular damage is the most likely cause, although myasthenia or early thyroid eye disease should never be excluded. Patients older than 50 are also at higher risk for temporal arteritis, which is potentially a blinding condition. The causes of new-onset double vision with both eyes open are shown in **Table 13.1**.

Cause of double vision	Symptoms
Microvascular	Painless; cardiovascular risk factors
Thyroid eye disease	Red eyes, history of thyroid disease; symptoms of hypo- or hyperthyroidism
Myasthenia	Varying double vision depending on the muscles affected Better after rest and worse at the end of the day More systemic features include ptosis and dysphagia
Trauma	There is a history of severe facial trauma/assault

Table 13.1 Common causes of new bilateral double vision

Further history

The patient explains that the double vision has been recent in onset and only occurs when both eyes are open. The two images are seen at an angle. The double vision seems to worsen at the end of the day. She has no other obvious weakness, but recently has had a slight difficulty in swallowing. She denies any history of trauma. There are no symptoms of temporal arteritis.

Previous medical history: The patient has mild hypertension.

Previous ocular history: The patient wears glasses for near reading.

Medications: The patient takes bendroflumethiazide for her hypertension.

Diagnostic approach

Examination, as always, should be thorough, initially looking to determine whether there are any external clues to the cause of diplopia, including ptosis and anisocoria in a third nerve palsy or hemiparesis in sixth and third nerve syndromes. This should be followed by a detailed examination of squint with the cover/uncover test, alternate cover test and ocular motility.

Examination

The examination shows nothing of note and there is no focal neurology.

Ophthalmic examination: The ophthalmic examination is summarised in **Table 13.2**.

Diagnostic approach

It is obvious that the weakness pattern is very variable and seems to be worse on retesting, indicating fatigability. This is highly indicative of myasthenia gravis. In addition, there seems to be a weakness of the inferior rectus and lateral rectus muscles. This makes a single nerve palsy unlikely as there would be a lateral rectus palsy and a partial third nerve palsy, which is highly unlikely.

Myasthenia can be tested for using the Tensilon (edrophonium) test, in which, under specialist supervision, edrophonium is administered to partially reverse any effects of myasthenia. The squint can then be remeasured during this time. In addition, a blood sample should be tested for anti-acetylcholine receptors;

Right eye		Left eye
6/6	**Visual acuity**	6/6
Normal direct and consensual reflex	**Pupil**	Normal direct and consensual reflex
Clear	**Cornea**	Clear
Clear	**Anterior chamber**	Clear
Clear	**Lens**	Clear
No movement when left covered	**Cover/uncover test**	Movement down and out when right covered
Marked vertical and horizontal movement	**Alternate cover test**	Marked vertical and horizontal movement
Full range of movement	**Ocular motility**	Reduced abduction and hypodeviation

Table 13.2 Ophthalmic examination: results for a patient who presented with new-onset double vision

this test is positive in over 95% of those with generalised myasthenia.

Different-sized pupils

Presentation

A 60-year-old man presents to his GP because of different-sized pupils (**anisocoria**), which he noticed when looking in the mirror.

Diagnostic approach

An understanding of what causes variation in pupil size helps to give a framework for the diagnosis. The history should cover possible localising signs for a difference in pupil size. However, it is the examination that will highlight which pupil is abnormal and that helps to differentiate the causes.

Diagnostic clues in the history: There are very few clues in the initial presentation. The patient's age makes it unlikely that an Adie pupil (tonic pupil) is the cause. **Table 13.3** lists possible clues in the history for anisocoria.

> ### Clinical insight
>
> A diagnosis of ocular myasthenia should always be kept as a differential in diplopia as it may mimic any palsy.

Causes of anisocoria	Possible clues in history
Physiological	Nil
Horner syndrome	Droopy eyelid; dry face; previous tumour in the brain, spine or lung; trauma to the neck; or headache from carotid artery dissection
Adie pupil	Younger female patient usually post viral
Argyll Robertson pupil	History of a rash on the hands and a gummatous growth on the body
Third nerve palsy	Double vision; droopy eyelid; headache if linked with aneurysm
Iritis	Photophobia; reduction in vision; red eye
Pharmacological	History of touching or using dilating or constricting drops
Trauma	History of knock to the eye

Table 13.3 Clues in the history for causes of anisocoria

Further history

The patient has had no headache or history of trauma and no double vision; he has no history of a previous tumour or surgery. He does, however, have a mildly droopy eyelid, and recently, he has also become increasingly wheezy and has occasionally noticed a tinge of blood in his cough.

Clinical insight

Generally, if the size difference is the same in the light as in the dark, this is likely to be physiological (<0.5 mm). If the difference is greater in light, then an Adie pupil is likely, whereas if the difference is greater in the dark, then a Horner pupil (sympathetic miosis) is far more likely.

Social history: The patient smokes 20 cigarettes a day

Diagnostic approach

Examination is the key to diagnosis. First, the eyes should be examined for ptosis or deviation. The pupil anisocoria should be measured in good lighting and then in the dark. Next, the direct and consensual reflex should be tested, followed by tests for a relative afferent pupillary defect. Finally, to test for light–near dissociation, the near response should be checked to see whether there is constriction.

Examination

The patient has a mild wheeze throughout both lung fields. There is dullness to percussion and auscultation at the left lung apex (**Figure 13.3**).

Ophthalmic examination: The ophthalmic examination is summarised in **Table 13.4**.

Diagnostic approach

The findings indicate Horner syndrome (oculosympathetic palsy). As a result, the patient's face should be tested further for anhidrosis and enophthalmos. The diagnosis can be confirmed using apraclonidine drops to both eyes; only the Horner pupil should dilate.

The level of dissociation can be confirmed by instilling 1% hydroxyamphetamine. A first- or second-order neurone

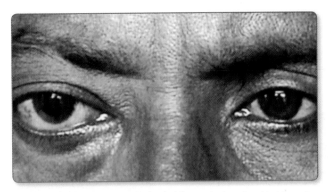

Figure 13.3 Patient who presented with different-sized pupils, with anisocoria and mild ptosis.

	Right eye		Left eye
	6/6	**Visual acuity**	6/6
	Normal direct and consensual reflex Normal near response	**Pupil**	Normal direct and consensual reflex Left pupil smaller than right and the difference increased with darkness. Normal near response
	Normal	**Lid**	Mild ptosis
	Full	**Ocular motility**	Full

Table 13.4 Ophthalmic examination: results for a patient who presented with different-sized pupils

abnormality will still result in dilation of the pupil whereas a third-order neurone defect will not. In this patient, a chest radiograph may be warranted because of haemoptysis, the smoking history and the abnormal respiratory examination (see **Figure 3.5**).

13.2 Third (oculomotor) nerve palsy

The third cranial nerve innervates the superior rectus, inferior rectus, medial rectus and inferior oblique muscles and, in so doing, controls elevation, depression and adduction of the eye. The nerve also innervates the levator palpebrae superioris, which controls lid elevation, and, via the associated parasympathetic nerves, the pupillary sphincter and ciliary body, thereby controlling pupil constriction and accommodation. The course of the oculomotor nerve is shown in **Figure 13.4**.

Guiding principle

A new oculomotor palsy may potentially result from life-threatening pathology. The most important sign to consider is whether the pupil is affected or spared. A new third nerve palsy that involves the pupil should undergo urgent neuroimaging investigation for a space-occupying lesion or posterior cerebellar communicating artery aneurysm.

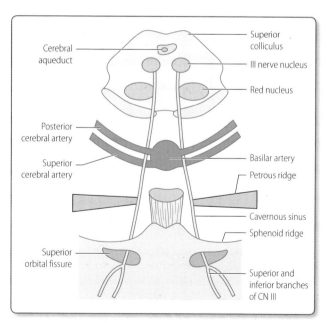

Figure 13.4 The course of the third cranial nerve.

Epidemiology
Third nerve palsy is a relatively rare condition.

Causes
The possible causes of third nerve palsy are shown in **Table 13.5**.

Pathogenesis
Third nerve insults can lead to either a complete or a partial third nerve palsy depending on the severity of the insult to the nerve. The palsy can also involve the pupil or be pupil sparing. The pupil-controlling parasympathetic fibres are found on the outside of the third nerve. Hence, pupil-involving third nerve palsies are likely to be more sinister compressive causes, such as an aneurysm or tumour. Non-pupil-affecting fibres are usually more central and are first to be affected by blockage to the **vaso nervorum**, i.e. small blood vessels supplying the nerves.

Anatomical location	Causes	Signs and symptoms
Nuclear	Infarction Haemorrhage Abscess Tumour	Bilateral ptosis Deficit in contralateral elevation
Midbrain	Infarction Haemorrhage Abscess Tumour	Possible ipsilateral ataxia, ipsilateral tremor or contralateral hemiparesis depending on site
Subarachnoid	Usually isolated	Aneurysm Infection
Cavernous sinus	Usually involves fourth and sixth nerve palsies	Microvascular infarction Carotid artery aneurysm/dissection Tumour
Orbital	Chemosis, proptosis Usually other cranial nerves	Inflammation Tumour

Table 13.5 Causes and clinical features of third nerve palsy by anatomical location

Clinical features

Patients with third nerve palsy have diplopia, which is both horizontal and vertical. The history should include any risk factors, especially for microvascular insult such as cardiovascular risk factors and age. Also, the history should include questions about any other associated neurological deficits. Third nerve palsy usually has some element of an elevation, depression and abduction defect associated with ptosis (**Figure 13.5**). **Table 13.5** lists other associated features that may provide a clue to anatomical location.

Investigations

Patients with painful third nerve palsies or pupil-involving third nerve palsies require an urgent MRI or MRI angiogram to exclude an intracranial aneurysm of the posterior communicating artery. Patients who have pupil-sparing third nerve palsies should be investigated for blood pressure, fasting glucose, erythrocyte sedimentation rate (ESR) and antineutrophil antibodies (ANAs) and should undergo Venereal Disease Research Laboratory (VDRL) tests. They may also require imaging if there is no resolution by 3 months or if they are younger than 50 years.

Differential diagnosis

For the differential diagnoses of diplopia, please see **Figure 3.3**.

Management

Management varies according to the cause. The majority of third nerve palsies are due to microvascular occlusion. The

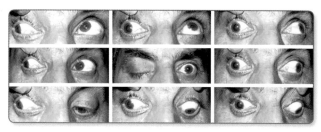

Figure 13.5 Right third nerve palsy in various positions of gaze.

majority of these resolve within 6 months and observation is key. Because of the vertical and horizontal nature of the double vision, the squint is often difficult to treat with prisms alone and occlusion is often required initially. For third nerve palsy that has remained stable for 6 months, surgery may be indicated.

Prognosis

The majority of cases are microangiopathic and resolve completely within 6 months.

13.3 Fourth (trochlear) nerve palsy

The fourth cranial nerve innervates the superior oblique muscle, which **intorts** (i.e. rotates the superior globe medially), depresses and abducts the globe. Fourth nerve palsy can be either congenital or acquired. The course of the fourth nerve is shown in **Figure 13.6**.

Epidemiology

Fourth nerve palsy is relatively rare, with peaks at birth owing to congenital fourth nerve palsy and in middle and late age

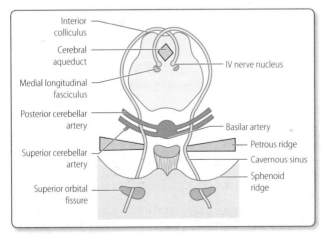

Figure 13.6 Course of the fourth cranial nerve.

owing to trauma and small vessel disease. It is less common than third or sixth cranial nerve palsy.

Causes

The causes of fourth cranial nerve palsy can be:

- traumatic
- microangiopathic as a result of damage to the fourth cranial nerve from secondary hypertension, diabetes or arteriosclerosis
- myasthenic
- congenital

Pathogenesis

Congenital fourth nerve palsy results from a dysgenesis of the fourth cranial nerve. The nerve dysgenesis has a corresponding tendon abnormality, which can be loose, incorrectly inserted or, occasionally, absent.

The fourth cranial nerve is susceptible to damage in trauma owing to its long course and close proximity to the tentorium, an extension of the dura that separates the cerebellum from the inferior portion of the cerebral hemispheres. Cavernous sinus pathology can also affect the fourth nerve, although other cranial nerves are usually also affected. Additionally, like other nerves, the fourth nerve is supplied by a vasa nervorum, which is susceptible to microangiopathic damage.

Clinical features

The most common symptom described by patients is vertical double vision. Double vision is worst in adduction and depression, and so activities such as reading and walking down stairs may exacerbate symptoms (see **Figure 13.7** for the eye movements that are affected). Unilateral fourth nerve palsy usually presents with patients who have a head tilt away from the side of the palsy in order to reduce diplopia. Very rarely in bilateral fourth nerve palsy, patients have a head-down position.

Differential diagnosis

The differential diagnoses of diplopia are shown in **Figure 3.3**.

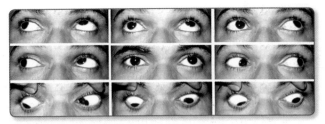

Figure 13.7 Fourth cranial nerve palsy in various positions of gaze.

Investigations

These should include blood pressure, fasting glucose, ESR, and ANAs and VDRL tests. They may also require imaging if there is no resolution by 3 months or if they are younger than 50 years.

Management

Microangiopathic cases can simply be observed. Prisms may be used to help small vertical deviations with few torsional symptoms. Surgical approaches to reduce vertical diplopia include a superior oblique tendon tuck in laxity. In congenital cases or contralateral inferior rectus weakening if there is no laxity.

In stable, acquired cases with small deviations and a duration >6 months, ipsilateral inferior oblique weakening can be used to reduce vertical deviation. With greater deviations, two or three muscles may have to be operated on in order to reduce deviation.

Prognosis

Patients with congenital palsy are able to accept greater vertical divergence than those with acquired palsy, hence not all patients require treatment. Treatment usually depends on whether a head posture is present. Acquired small vessel disease usually resolves within 6 months.

13.4 Sixth (abducent) nerve palsy

The sixth cranial nerve innervates the ipsilateral lateral rectus. The nucleus is located in the pons just medial to the facial nerve nucleus. It travels along the floor of the lateral ventricle and enters the subarachnoid space when it emerges from the brainstem. The nerve then runs upward between the pons and the clivus, and then pierces the dura to run between the dura and the skull, making a sharp turn at the petrous temporal bone and clivus to enter the cavernous sinus. In the cavernous sinus, it runs alongside the internal carotid artery before entering the orbit through the superior orbital fissure and innervating the lateral rectus muscle of the eye (**Figure 13.8**).

Epidemiology

In adults, the sixth cranial nerve is the most commonly affected of the cranial nerves innervating motor functions in the eye. In children, it is the second most commonly affected (after the fourth cranial nerve).

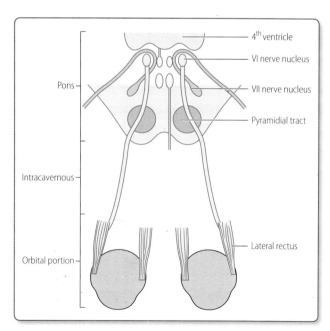

Figure 13.8 Course of the sixth cranial nerve.

Causes

The causes of sixth cranial nerve palsy can be:

- idiopathic
- microangiopathic
- due to raised intracranial pressure
- due to a tumour
- due to meningitis
- due to a carotid cavernous fistula

Pathogenesis

The sixth cranial nerve has a long course, and disruption can occur as a result of anatomical relations along its path. At the pons, the facial nerve is also usually affected because of the proximity of the two nuclei, commonly caused by demyelination and tumours. Raised intracranial pressure can force the brainstem to be pushed down and therefore stretch the nerve along the clivus. Intracavernous carotid aneurysms can cause compression. Additionally, the vasa nervorum can be occluded.

Clinical features

Patients have horizontal double vision that worsens on gaze to the side of the deficit and to the distance. Other neurological symptoms may provide information about the anatomical location (**Table 13.6**). Examination reveals reduced abduction on the side of the abnormality (**Figure**

Anatomical location	Signs
Dorsal pons	Ipsilateral gaze loss OR Contralateral hemiparesis OR Ipsilateral facial nerve palsy
Dorsolateral pons	Ipsilateral trigeminal and facial nerve loss and contralateral hemianaesthesia

Table 13.6 Anatomical clues to the site of a lesion from examination of sixth nerve palsy

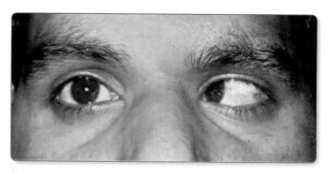

Figure 13.9 Left sixth cranial nerve palsy.

13.9) and, occasionally, a head posture towards the affected eye. In severe palsies, the eyes may even be convergent in normal gaze.

Investigations

Blood pressure, glucose and cholesterol should be checked for microangiopathic risk factors. A blood sample for a full blood count, ESR and C-reactive protein level should be taken to exclude temporal arteritis.

Differential diagnosis

The differential diagnoses of sixth cranial nerve palsy include the following (see also **Figure 3.3**):

- restrictive disease such as Duane syndrome (eye retraction syndrome)
- thyroid eye disease
- chronic progressive external ophthalmoplegia

Management

Microangiopathic sixth nerve palsy can be treated conservatively to check for resolution. If the sixth nerve palsy is partial, a prism may be fitted to glasses or botox can be administered to weaken the medial rectus. Other options include lateral rectus resection and medial rectus recession if the findings are stable for at least 6 months. Complete sixth nerve palsy requires the position of the superior and inferior rectus muscles to be moved to assist eye movement if prisms are ineffective.

Prognosis

The most common cause is microangiopathic palsy, and this usually resolves by 6 months. Further investigation is needed for more sinister causes if there is no resolution by 3 months or if patients are younger than 50.

13.5 Non-paralytic squints

A non-paralytic or concomitant squint is one in which the angle between the eyes remains constant in all angles of gaze. Non-paralytic squints are most commonly divided into squints in which the angle is convergent (**esodeviation**) and those in which the angle is divergent (**exodeviation**). They are commonly found in childhood.

> ### Guiding principle
>
> Squints in children are especially important to diagnose and treat early as they may lead to amblyopia, i.e. irreversible loss of vision due to the failure of processing.

Epidemiology

Non-paralytic squints are relatively common in children, with up to 5% affected.

Pathogenesis

Unlike paralytic strabismus, the efferent pathways are intact in concomitant or non-paralytic strabismus, but there is an abnormality in fusion and fixation that is thought to be central. Non-paralytic strabismus may also occur as a result of differences in the eyes, e.g. secondary to refractive power differences, media opacity such as cataract or abnormal retinal image localisation. Finally, high hypermetropia may result in an accommodative response causing the eyes to converge.

Clinical features

Usually, the squint is noted by parents or teachers of the child. Further questioning may elucidate the type of squint. The history should include when the squint occurs, the refractive status and the visual status of the child if known. Other background information includes birth, previous medical and family history.

The first aim of examination should be to determine whether this is a true squint. Occasionally, epicanthal folds or asymmetry can mimic a squint. The child should be refracted and the visual acuity tested before the squint is measured using the cover/uncover test and the alternate cover test; the ocular movements should also be examined. Finally, a full dilated fundal examination is used to exclude intraocular pathology.

Differential diagnosis

The differential diagnoses for diplopia are shown in **Figure 3.3**.

Management

The first aim is to correct any refractive error fully. Sometimes, strabismus can completely resolve with this treatment. Amblyopia (see Chapter 14) may need to be treated by drops or patching to the non-amblyopic eye. Finally, surgery may be required to realign the eyes, with a resection or advancement to strengthen muscle power and recession to weaken muscles.

Prognosis

The prognosis is usually good with regards to vision if any amblyopia can be treated early. However, children tend to lose binocular vision early.

13.6 Nystagmus

Nystagmus is a repetitive, rhythmic, involuntary movement of the eyes. Most commonly, it is horizontal, but it may also be vertical or torsional. Jerk-type nystagmus is described by the direction of movement of the fast phase.

Causes

The causes of nystagmus can be:

- physiological: found on extremes of gaze
- congenital: inherited or secondary to poor vision
- due to drugs/toxicity
- due to focal neurological disease, e.g. a space-occupying lesions, demyelination, cerebrovascular disease or trauma

Pathogenesis

A stable eye position is used to maintain images on the fovea. The position is maintained by a complex interaction between the eye and the vestibular system. Defects in any of these pathways may result in nystagmus.

Clinical features

Patients with nystagmus may have vertigo or the feeling that the world is constantly moving (i.e. oscillopsia). Patients may find that certain positions of gaze can reduce this sensation (this is known as the null point). Further questioning can include that of family, birth, drug, occupational and social history.

Examination should include a description of the nystagmus. A useful mnemonic is DWARF, i.e. **d**irection, **w**aveform, **a**mplitude, **r**educing **d**irection, **f**requency – and a full examination of vision and ocular motility.

Congenital nystagmus commonly has a pendular pattern, with equal speed of eye movement in either direction. Other clues to the anatomical location can be found from the description (**Table 13.7**). Other examination should include vision, which is usually reduced in congenital nystagmus, and a full ocular motility examination.

Investigations

New nystagmus usually requires MRI imaging to exclude sinister intracerebral pathology.

Management

Toxic substances or drugs inducing nystagmus should be avoided. For patients with congenital nystagmus, full refractive

Type of nystagmus	Anatomical clue
Jerk	Cerebellar
Down for fast beat	Foramen magnum lesion, e.g. Arnold–Chiari malformation (cerebellomedullary malformation syndrome)
Up for fast beat	Brainstem
See-saw	Chiasmal lesion
Convergence retraction nystagmus, i.e. nystagmus on upgaze resulting from repeated convergence	Dorsal midbrain

Table 13.7 Anatomical clues to the site of lesions from the description of nystagmus

correction should be given to improve vision. Gabapentin can be used to reduce symptoms in congenital nystagmus by slowing the rate of oscillation.

Finally, if a null point is observed, prisms can be used to force the gaze towards the null point and hence reduce amplitude.

Prognosis

Nystagmus is rarely completely cured except in cases resulting from vestibular and demyelinating causes.

13.7 Pupil disorders

Pupil dilatation is controlled by the sympathetic pathway, and constriction by the parasympathetic pathway. Anisocoria is the term used to describe asymmetric pupils (**Figures 13.1** and **13.2**).

Epidemiology

Up to 20% of people have physiologic anisocoria.

Causes

The causes of anisocoria are shown in **Table 13.8**.

Smaller pupil	Larger pupil
Physiological	Physiological
Horner syndrome	Adie pupil
Argyll Robertson pupil	Trauma
Old Adie syndrome	Sympathomimetic drops, e.g. tropicamide
Parasympathomimetic drops	Third nerve palsy
Anterior uveitis	

Table 13.8 Causes of small and large pupils

Pathogenesis
Anisocoria results most commonly from a disruption to either the pupil constrictive or pupil dilatory pathways.

Clinical features
The clinical features are summarised in **Table 13.9**.

Investigations
The investigations are summarised in **Table 13.9**.

Differential diagnosis
For the differential diagnoses of anisocoria, see **Figure 3.5**.

Management
The management is summarised in **Table 13.9**.

Condition	Symptoms	Signs	Investigations	Treatment
Horner syndrome	Dry face; history of smoking with lung cancer or trauma	Mild ptosis, anhidrosis, enophthalmos with miosis. Pupil dilates following instillation of apraclonidine	New Horner syndrome requires chest radiograph to exclude upper lobe lung tumour and MRI to exclude spinal or midbrain pathology. If the patient has pain/headache, an MR angiogram is used to exclude carotid artery dissection	Treatment of underlying cause
Argyll Robertson pupil	History of syphilis or other non-specific neurology	Occasionally, chorioretinitis. Other signs of tertiary syphilis, including aortitis and tabes dorsalis	Syphilis serology	Liaise closely with genitourinary team Intramuscular penicillin
Anterior uveitis	Painful red photophobic eye	Cells in the anterior chamber and fixed pupil with adhesions on dilation	See Chapter 10 for more details	See Chapter 10 for more details
Adie pupil	Blurring of vision; occasionally post viral. Mainly in young women	Reacts very slowly to light but more briskly to a near response. May be associated with abnormal reflexes in Holmes–Adie syndrome	Pilocarpine 0.1% is instilled in both eyes. Only an Adie pupil will constrict owing to denervation hypersensitivity	Pilocarpine used for cosmesis
Third nerve palsy	Double vision. Previous history of diabetes or hypertension in arteriopathic cases	Marked ptosis, with the eye down and out and usually a fixed and dilated pupil if the palsy is complete	A new pupil-affecting third nerve palsy requires urgent MRI or MR angiogram to exclude a new posterior cerebral artery aneurysm	Neurosurgical opinion for either clipping or coiling of the aneurysm

Table 13.9 Symptoms, signs, investigation and treatments for various causes of anisocoria

Paediatric ophthalmology

In terms of years of life affected by vision, the childhood eye diseases are the most relevant. The majority of diseases are, however, treatable and reversible if diagnosed early. The difficulty is examining young patients who are unable to properly describe their symptoms. Therefore, the eye examination is particularly important. The visual tests need to be tailored to the age and stage of development of the patient. Screening programmes have also been organised in developed countries for many of these conditions.

Embryology

The eye begins to develop early in foetal life as an outgrowth from the primitive forebrain, and is virtually complete in structure by a fetal age of about 3 months. At full term, the anatomical elements are almost complete; however, the iris is yet to be fully pigmented and the accommodation apparatus remains relatively underdeveloped. The visual processing pathways continue to develop and remain plastic until about 8 years old.

14.1 Clinical scenario

Absent red reflex

Presentation

A 2-year-old girl presents to the ophthalmic outpatients department because her parents have noticed that she has no red reflex on photographs and has a slight whitening of the pupil on the right.

Diagnostic approach

Loss of the red reflex is a relatively common presentation to a paediatric eye clinic. There should be a low threshold for specialist referral. There are several causes for loss of the red reflex, the most common of which is bilateral loss in darker skinned individuals. However, a whitening of the pupil (i.e. **leukocoria**) may have more serious consequences. The history from the parents' observations is important in children, but the examination is key.

The presentation provides little clue to the cause.

Further history

The child has been otherwise well with no recent illness. She has reached all relevant milestones, and her vaccinations are up to date.

Family history: The patient's father was treated as a child for an eye tumour.

Previous ocular history: There is no previous ocular history of note for the patient. Her red reflex was normal at the 6-week baby check, and her vision was fine at 8 months old.

Diagnostic approach

The patient should be examined with full dilatation, looking at the eye from front to back.

Examination

There is nothing of note in the examination.

Ophthalmic examination: The ophthalmic examination is summarised in **Table 14.1**.

Diagnostic approach

The examination has confirmed a large white growth in the retina. This requires urgent specialist tertiary referral for diagnosis and early treatment. Obviously, careful counselling is required. From the family history, timing and appearance, this is highly likely to be retinoblastoma. The other differential diagnoses of leukocoria are shown in **Table 14.2**.

14.2 Amblyopia

Amblyopia is reduced vision in an eye without ocular pathology that cannot be completely improved by refractive correction. It can be unilateral and, less commonly, bilateral.

	Right eye		Left eye
Visual acuity	Only seeing hand movements in the periphery		6/6 on Kay picture test cards
Pupil	No direct or consensual reflex Right relative afferent pupillary defect		Normal direct and consensual reflex
Cornea	Clear		Clear
Anterior chamber	Clear		Clear
Lens	Clear		Clear
Vitreous	Clear		Clear
Retina	Large exophytic white growth		Clear

Table 14.1 Ophthalmic examination: results for a patient who presented with absent red reflex

Cause	Description
Cataract	Needs to be treated as soon as possible to avoid amblyopia
Persistent hyperplastic primary vitreous	Remains of the early foetal vasculature
Retinoblastoma	Malignant disease of primitive retinal cells
Coats disease (exudative retinitis)	Exudation of creamy material from telangiectatic vessels; more common in boys
Retinopathy of prematurity	Abnormal vessel growth and retinal detachment in those born before 32 weeks gestation and weighing <1500 g
Coloboma	Whitening showing the sclera as a result of incomplete closure of the eye during embryogenesis
Toxocara	Infectious granuloma caused by a nematode whose definitive hosts are dogs

Table 14.2 Differential diagnoses of leukocoria

Epidemiology

Amblyopia has a cumulative incidence of 2–4% in children up to the age of 16. There is an increased incidence in those who are born prematurely or developmentally delayed.

Causes

The causes of amblyopia include:
- refractive error
- anisometropia (a difference in the refractive power between the eyes)
- squint
- obstruction to vision, e.g. cataract, ptosis or corneal scarring

Pathogenesis

Amblyopia is a developmental abnormality rather than an organic pathology. The differential input to both the fovea and retina mean that the brain, which shows great plasticity in the early years, suppresses binocular processing to allow a single visual input. Conflicting images, such as from a squint, anisometropia or block to the visual axis of one eye, are stimulating factors for this process. However, poor vision in both eyes may result in bilateral amblyopia. It is thought that the risk remains until the age of 7 or 8, with onset more profound and more rapid at a younger age.

Clinical features

It is important in the history to ask about pathological causes of loss of vision, such as surgery or trauma. In addition, it is useful to ask for other risks, including birth history and developmental delay. Amblyopia can be diagnosed by looking at visual acuity: there is a greater than two-line difference in vision that is sometimes worsened by placing the letters close to each other, known as the crowding phenomenon. Examination should include a full dilated fundoscopic examination to exclude intraocular pathology along with a cycloplegic refraction to check for refractive error. Squints should be evaluated by orthoptists.

Investigations

If there is any doubt about the organic pathology, MRI of the head is indicated.

Differential diagnosis

The differential diagnoses include those in **Figure 3.2**.

Management

The aims of good management of amblyopia are to identify those with, or who are at high risk for, amblyopia early in order to minimise the visual deficit. This is usually achieved by childhood screening programmes for vision at 6 weeks (checking the red reflex) and 8 months (brief vision check) and early referral. Any pathology such as ptosis or cataract should be operated on swiftly to prevent worsening of amblyopia.

Children should have full refractive correction to minimise any anisometropia. Lack of improvement or dense amblyopia then warrants occlusion or penalisation therapy. Occlusion therapy involves placing a patch over the 'good' eye to encourage the brain to upregulate the 'poor' eye. Penalisation therapy uses atropine drops to blur the 'good' eye for similar effect.

Prognosis

If treatment has not occurred by the age of 7 or 8, recovery is extremely unlikely, although there is some evidence that slower recovery can still occur until the age of 12. With treatment, approximately one quarter of children improve.

14.3 Retinopathy of prematurity

Retinopathy of prematurity (ROP) is a retinal vessel developmental disorder that affects children born before 32 weeks gestation and who weigh <1500 g at birth.

Epidemiology

Approximately 50% of infants who weigh <1500 g at birth and who are born at <32 weeks gestation develop ROP. The lower the gestational age and weight at birth, the greater the risk. ROP is slightly more common among boys and those from Caucasian populations.

Pathogenesis

The eye blood vessels begin to grow from the putative optic nerve at approximately week 6 of gestation, completing their growth just after birth. However, if a child is born prematurely, this growth is incomplete. It is thought that tissue in the periphery of the retina releases several growth factors, including transforming growth factor and vascular endothelial growth factor, that result in misdirected growth of the vasculature, causing ROP. There are various stages of ROP, from minor vessel changes including tortuosity to abnormal fronds of growth, traction and retinal detachment. Other complications in later life include amblyopia, myopia and glaucoma.

Clinical features

Children within the age and weight criteria for ROP are now screened weekly in developed countries for ROP. In developing countries, children who have not been screened may present when the parents notice that the child has reduced vision, squint or loss of the red reflex. Children should be screened with full dilated fundoscopy and an indirect ophthalmoscope or with a special wide angle retinal camera.

Diagnostic criteria

The diagnostic criteria include:

Stage I: mildly abnormal blood vessel growth. Many children who develop stage I improve with no treatment and eventually develop normal vision

Stage II: moderately abnormal blood vessel growth. Many children who develop stage II improve with no treatment and eventually develop normal vision

Stage III: severely abnormal blood vessel growth. The abnormal blood vessels grow towards the centre of the eye instead of following their normal growth pattern along the surface of the retina. Some infants who develop stage III improve with no treatment and eventually develop normal vision. However, treatment should be considered for those children who have thicker and more tortuous blood vessels, known as plus disease (**Figure 14.1**)

Stage IV: partially detached retina. Traction from scarring produced by bleeding of abnormal vessels pulls the retina away from the wall of the eye

Stage V: completely detached retina and the end-stage of the disease.

Differential diagnosis

The differential diagnoses include:

- persistent hyperplastic primary vitreous
- exudative retinal disease

Management

Management varies as to the staging of the disease. Usually, stage I, II and III disease can be observed. Active stage III

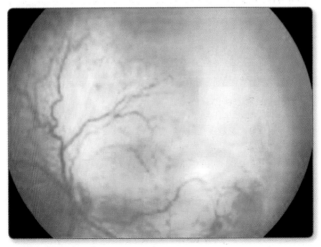

Figure 14.1 Retinopathy of prematurity showing a vascular ridge.

should be treated with cryotherapy or laser to the region peripheral to the vessel development. Stage IV and V disease require retinal surgery with a peripheral buckle or vitreous surgery.

Prognosis

Despite advances in screening and treatment, retinal detachment is thought to occur in around 10% of eyes.

14.4 Retinoblastoma

Retinoblastoma is a childhood ocular cancer originating from primitive retinal cells.

Epidemiology

Retinoblastoma is the most common ocular tumour in childhood. It affects approximately 1 in 18,000 children under the age of 5. The incidence is higher in developing countries.

Pathogenesis

Retinoblastoma results from either sporadic or inherited mutations in the retinoblastoma gene 13q. Retinoblastoma follows the Knudson two-hit model, in which both of the alleles of the protective gene need to be mutated or lost from a cell for retinoblastoma to develop.

In the sporadic form, both mutational events occur within a cell after fertilisation. In the inherited form, one mutation is inherited in all cells and the other occurs after birth. Those with inherited forms of the condition are at very high risk of developing retinoblastoma; common forms include multifocal, bilateral and trilateral. Other non-ocular tumours can occur, such as pineoblastoma of the pineal gland.

Clinical features

In the developed world, retinoblastoma most commonly presents as leukocoria, i.e. whitening of the pupil and loss of the red reflex (**Figure 14.2**). More rarely, examination can reveal strabismus, anterior chamber cells or **pseudohypopyon**, a fluid level in the anterior chamber and proptosis. Dilated fundus

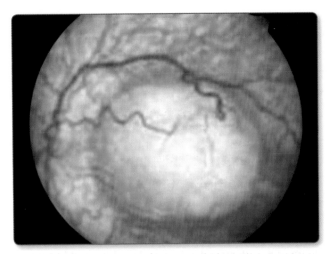

Figure 14.2 Retinoblastoma.

examination reveals a creamy, whitened lesion and retinal detachment.

Investigations

Ultrasound can be used to diagnose a tumour if the fundal view is not clear. CT can also aid diagnosis because of intraocular calcification; MRI can be used to delineate extension into the optic nerve and to demonstrate the presence of any related intracerebral pathology. Biopsy increases the risk of metastatic disease, but enucleation is still used in equivocal cases in which vision has already been affected.

Differential diagnosis

The differential diagnoses include:
- Coats disease (exudative retinitis): this is usually unilateral with telangiectatic blood vessels
- Toxocara: there is an abscess in the retina
- persistent primary hyperplastic vitreous: there are remnants of the hyaloid artery that ran from the optic nerve to the lens during foetal life

Management

Management is multidisciplinary, and involves ophthalmologists, oncologists, paediatricians, genetic counsellors and radiotherapists. A variety of treatment modalities are available, including thermotherapy, brachytherapy, chemotherapy, cryotherapy, laser and enucleation. Measures vary as to the staging of treatment.

Prognosis

Retinoblastoma can be life threatening once there is extraocular spread. Screening should occur during the early years for those with inherited retinoblastoma. Early detection facilitates purely intraocular treatment, which can potentially salvage both the eye and vision. Most children, however, have relatively advanced disease and require enucleation, which has a 95% cure rate.

Eye injuries account for a considerable proportion of avoidable pain, distress and loss of vision.

The key to detecting sight-threatening trauma is to adopt a high degree of suspicion that an occult serious injury may underlie seemingly innocuous superficial manifestations of injury. The true nature of an injury is revealed through a routine of detailed history, visual acuity, visual fields, pupil responses and signs of injury around the eye and elsewhere in the body.

15.1 Clinical scenario

Squash ball injury of the eye

Presentation

A 34-year-old man presents to the emergency department after having a squash ball strike his right eye.

Diagnostic approach

In the history, it is important to ascertain the mechanism of any injury to provide information about possible damage and any deficit the patient has noticed. However, thorough examination is key, along with documentation for possible medicolegal reasons.

Diagnostic clues in the history: The size of a squash ball means that it is unlikely that the eye would be fully protected from the force of the injury by the bony orbit; hence, there should be a high level of suspicion for an ocular injury and blow-out fractures of the orbital bones.

Further history

The patient feels that his vision is reduced in the right eye. He does not have any double vision; however, there is a continued dull ache with foreign body sensation.

Diagnostic approach

There should be a detailed examination of the eye from the orbit and lids to the back.

Examination

Ophthalmic examination: There is no obvious tenderness of the orbital bones, no lid laceration and the sensation to the infraorbital nerve is intact. There is bruising and swelling of the lid. There is no obvious deviation of the eyes with full ocular movement.

The remaining ophthalmic examination is summarised in **Table 15.1**.

Diagnostic approach

It appears that there is blood in the anterior chamber (**hyphaema**), in addition to an abrasion. This may account for the loss of vision.

Right eye		Left eye
Hand movements Hand movements	**Visual acuity** **Distance unaided** **Pinhole**	6/6 6/6
Pupil dilated with no direct but consensual reflex No RAPD	**Pupil**	Normal direct and no consensual reflex No RAPD
Abrasion highlighted by fluorescein	**Cornea**	Clear
Blood filled; difficult to see the pupil	**Anterior chamber**	Clear
No clear view	**Lens**	Clear
Unable to see clearly	**Vitreous**	Clear
Poor view of fundus	**Fundus**	Clear view of fundus
Difficult to view	**Disc**	Normal vessels and disc
RAPD, relative afferent pupillary defect.		

Table 15.1 Ophthalmic examination: results for a patient who presented with a squash ball injury

To confirm this, an ultrasound can be performed to rule out vitreous haemorrhage or retinal detachment. It is a good sign that there is no relative afferent pupillary defect (RAPD), which indicates that the optic nerve has not been affected. Treatment for this patient should in clude bed rest. Also, cyclopentolate 1% should be given three times a day to paralyse the iris, and dexamethasone should be instilled four times a day to reduce the risk of inflammation.

The patient should be reviewed daily for progression and for intraocular pressure, which can spike as a result of blood occluding the trabecular meshwork.

15.2 Chemical injury

Chemical eye injury can occur from any exogenous chemical administered to the eye or surrounding skin and is an ophthalmic emergency.

Epidemiology
The majority of chemical eye injuries occur in the workplace, followed by domestic incidents and finally assault cases. Men are more commonly afflicted than women.

Causes
The types of chemical that can cause injury include:
- cleaning products, e.g. bleach
- industrial acids or alkalis
- cement or plaster
- battery acid
- cosmetics

Pathogenesis
The most important feature to distinguish is whether the chemical was acid or alkali. The mechanism of damage differs with the type of injury. Acid injury is mainly a superficial

Guiding principle
This is an ophthalmic emergency. The aim is to institute immediate management to wash out and neutralise chemicals with water. There should be no delay in order to take a detailed history or to carry out an examination. Later treatment for damage and to assist healing can be applied once in the hospital setting if required.

disease as **coagulative necrosis** occurs, which prevents further penetration of chemical beyond the cornea. Alkali injury causes a disruptive **liquefactive necrosis** with breakdown of normal cellular barriers, facilitating deeper penetration of chemicals.

Clinical features

Patients usually describe a splash of chemical followed by associated symptoms, including:

- pain
- redness
- watering
- foreign body sensation
- reduced vision

It is important to ask about the type of chemical, as this could affect prognosis and further management, and whether irrigation has already been carried out. Examination should be systematic and include:

- vision
- conjunctival examination: redness or blanching (**Figure 15.1**)
- an assessment of limbal vessel loss

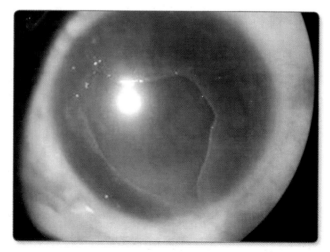

Figure 15.1 Chemical injury with limbal ischaemia and corneal haze.

- fornix examination: including the area of conjunctiva between the lids and the globe for injury and residual chemical
- assessment of the corneal epithelium and stroma
- an intraocular pressure check
- an assessment of the anterior chamber for inflammation
- fluorescein stain to reveal the presence of **punctate epithelial defects**, small circumscribed loss of the epithelium or complete epithelial loss

Diagnostic criteria
A simple method of classifying the severity of chemical injury is the Roper-Hall classification (**Table 15.2**).

Investigations
The pH should be tested with graduated Litmus paper to check for deviation from neutral. This should be checked regularly, even after irrigation, as there may be residual chemical.

Differential diagnosis
The differential diagnoses include:
- *allergic conjunctivitis*: this usually causes itch
- *corneal abrasion*: there is a history of abrasion rather than chemical injury

Grade	Appearance of cornea	Blanching of limbal vessels	Prognosis
I	Clear	Nil	Good
II	Hazy but iris details visible	<1/3	Good
III	Opaque cornea. Iris details obscured and total epithelial loss	1/3 to 1/2	Guarded
IV	Cornea opaque with pupil obscured	>1/2	Poor

Table 15.2 The Roper-Hall classification of chemical injury. Adapted from Roper-Hall MJ. Thermal and chemical burns. *Trans Ophthalmol Soc UK* 1965;85:631–53.

Clinical insight

A good way to check if pH has returned to normal is by checking against the unaffected eye.

Management

This consists of immediate management to reduce damage and intermediate management to promote healing. Late management is applied to correct any secondary damage.

Immediate management

Immediate management is to:
- wash the eye thoroughly with water and continue until the pH returns to normal or for a prolonged period if no pH reading is possible
- evert the lids as this is a common area for chemicals such as plaster to be retained
- wait to take a detailed history: it is more important to wash the eye

Intermediate management

Intermediate management includes topical antibiotics (preservative-free chloramphenicol four times a day) and lubricants (preservative-free carmellose four times a day and liquid paraffin at night).

For more severe injuries, topical preservative-free corticosteroids (prednisolone 0.5% four times a day), oral vitamin C (1 g twice a day) and oral doxycycline (100 mg twice a day) to reduce scarring are prescribed.

Late treatment

Late treatment includes that for limbal cell loss (limbal stem cell transplantation), fornix disruption (conjunctival reconstruction) and corneal scarring (corneal transplant).

Prognosis

The prognosis is worse for alkali injuries, injuries in which there has been a marked aberration from normal pH and a prolonged exposure to a chemical.

15.3 Corneal foreign body

Epidemiology

This is a common presentation to the emergency department. This most commonly occurs in young men, especially those in certain occupations such as welding or joinery.

Causes

Corneal foreign bodies can consist of:

* metal
* plastic
* glass
* sand

Pathogenesis

Foreign bodies occur commonly in the workplace or when wind blows dust or debris into the eye. The foreign body can either be embedded in the epithelium or in deeper layers if the foreign body has entered with any great velocity. Superficial foreign bodies can be removed by the upper lid, leading to a subtarsal foreign body that causes recurrent abrasion of the cornea. If the foreign body is not removed, there is an increased risk of infection or localised granulomatous inflammation in the case of metal foreign bodies.

Clinical features

The clinical features may include:

* grittiness or a foreign body sensation
* tearing
* photophobia
* a reduction in vision
* redness

Examination may reveal the foreign body or other sequelae, such as a rust ring or early infection. Long-standing irritation may lead to anterior

Clinical insight

Have a low suspicion for foreign bodies entering the eye. Usually these can be ruled out by examination for possible entry points, lateral X-ray for metals or orbital CT scan.

chamber inflammation. If not seen clearly, fluorescein can be used. Examination is also not complete without everting the lid to check for a subtarsal foreign body.

Differential diagnosis
It must be remembered that any corneal irritation can result in foreign body sensation even in the absence of an actual foreign body. Differential diagnoses include::
- keratitis
- dry eyes
- corneal abrasion

Management
An attempt at foreign body removal should be made, following instillation of topical anaesthetic (e.g. oxybuprocaine 0.4%). Patients should be aligned on the slit lamp and asked to focus in a particular direction. A sterile 21-gauge needle can then be used to remove the foreign body.

Prognosis
The prognosis is usually good unless the foreign body is central, or there is associated infection or inflammation. Patients with work-related foreign bodies should be counselled to wear fully protective glasses in the future.

15.4 Penetrating trauma

Penetrating trauma describes any injury that leads to open communication between the external environment and the inside of the eye.

Clinical insight

Always have a low threshold for suspecting penetrating injury to the eye as missed intraocular penetration or foreign bodies can lead to severe infection or inflammation.

Epidemiology
The incidence of penetrating eye injury is relatively rare. The incidence of penetrating intraocular foreign body is <0.2 cases per 100,000, with the majority of cases being young males. The number

of cases of penetrating trauma have reduced following the compulsory wearing of seatbelts.

Causes
The causes of penetrating trauma include:
- hammering
- glass
- knife injuries
- darts/arrows/airguns
- plants

Pathogenesis
The main barriers to penetration are the cornea anteriorly and sclera peripherally. Breach of these structures leads to a penetrating injury.

Clinical features
As these are often sensitive medicolegal cases, a thorough history and examination with comprehensive legible documentation is important. The history should include the nature of the materials and the mechanism of possible penetration. Patients should be asked about their tetanus status. Any possibility of a high-velocity injury, e.g. hammering metal, should lead to suspicion of an intraocular foreign body.

> **Clinical insight**
>
> Examination should be carried out carefully with little pressure placed on the eye in order to prevent prolapse of the intraocular contents. This is helped by the application of topical anaesthesia if the patient is unable to keep the eyelids open.

Vision and pupil reflexes, including the presence or absence of a RAPD, should be documented thoroughly. Penetrating trauma may lead to damage to any structure, e.g. corneal laceration, hyphaema, a distorted pupil, traumatic cataract, vitreous haemorrhage, retinal detachment and prolapsed intraocular contents.

Investigations
The primary aim of investigations is to search for intraocular foreign body, using:

- radiographs
- CT of the orbits

Note that MRI is not used initially in case the foreign body is metallic.

Management

If penetrating injury is noted, specialist care is required. The patient should be kept rested, nil by mouth and a shield placed over the eye. The patient should also be vaccinated against tetanus if indicated, and should be given analgesia.

Specialised treatment is usually undertaken in the operating theatre. If foreign bodies are not noted or are not easily accessible, a primary closure is undertaken. Intraocular foreign body, vitreous haemorrhage or retinal detachment may require further specialised vitreoretinal surgical intervention. Postoperative high-dose oral antibiotics (ciprofloxacin 750 mg twice a day), frequent corticosteroid drops (dexamethasone four times a day) and topical antibiotics (ofloxacin four times a day) should be administered.

Prognosis

The most important prognostic indicators are initial vision and RAPD. Loss of RAPD gives a very poor prognosis.

15.5 Blunt orbital trauma

This describes non-penetrating, high-impact trauma to the eye and surrounding structures (**Figure 15.2**).

Epidemiology

This occurs more commonly in young males. The number of cases of blunt trauma have reduced following the compulsory wearing of seatbelts.

Causes

The causes of blunt orbital trauma include:
- sports
- assault
- accident

Pathogenesis

The orbit is an enclosed box with the only outlet being anteriorly. The orbital rim is able to protect the globe from the majority of large objects, although there may be bruising or fracture to the bones in the process. Objects smaller than the orbital opening, e.g. a squash ball, may directly damage the globe. This results in increased intraorbital pressure and potentially globe damage.

Compression and decompression may result in intraocular damage by producing marked shearing forces (see below); in addition, the increased intraorbital pressure may result in a blow-out fracture, causing entrapment of the intraorbital contents including the extraocular muscles.

Clinical features

It is important to understand the mechanism to obtain information about the injuries.

Patients most commonly have:

- pain
- swelling
- reduced vision

Less commonly, they may have double vision.

Documentation should legibly state examination of:

- vision
- pupil reactions, including for a RAPD
- cornea and sclera for signs of rupture
- anterior chamber for deepening or hyphaema
- iris for traumatic mydriasis
- lens for cataract or abnormal movement
- vitreous for haemorrhage
- retina for detachment, commotio retinae (i.e. post-traumatic whitening caused by a sheared neuroretina), choroidal rupture
- optic nerve for optic neuropathy or swelling
- orbit for signs of fracture, crepitus and inferior orbital nerve sensation on the cheek below the eye
- eyes for enophthalmos and ocular movements

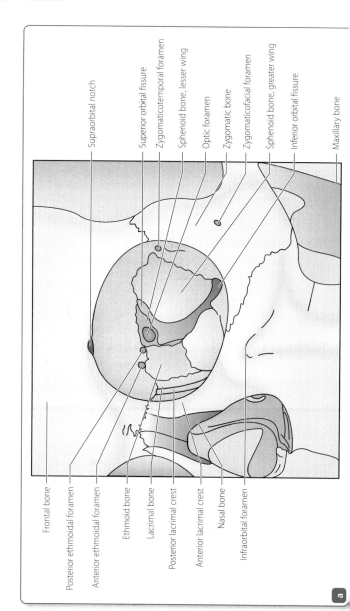

Supraorbital notch
Superior orbital fissure
Zygomaticotemporal foramen
Sphenoid bone, lesser wing
Optic foramen
Zygomatic bone
Zygomaticofacial foramen
Sphenoid bone, greater wing
Inferior orbital fissure
Maxillary bone

Frontal bone
Posterior ethmoidal foramen
Anterior ethmoidal foramen
Ethmoid bone
Lacrimal bone
Posterior lacrimal crest
Anterior lacrimal crest
Nasal bone
Infraorbital foramen

a

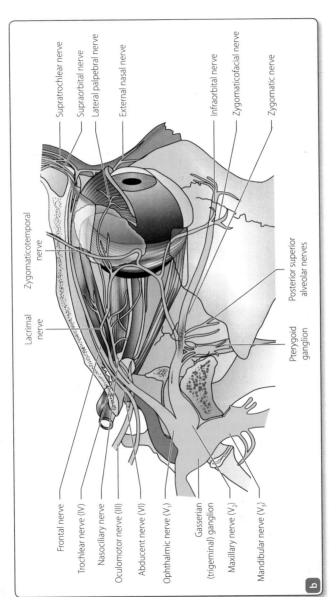

Figure 15.2 (a) The orbital bones. (b) The infraorbital nerve.

Supratrochlear nerve

Supraorbital nerve

Lateral palpebral nerve

External nasal nerve

Infraorbital nerve

Zygomaticofacial nerve

Zygomatic nerve

Zygomaticotemporal nerve

Lacrimal nerve

Posterior superior alveolar nerves

Pterygoid ganglion

Frontal nerve

Trochlear nerve (IV)

Nasociliary nerve

Oculomotor nerve (III)

Abducent nerve (VI)

Ophthalmic nerve (V₁)

Gasserian (trigeminal) ganglion

Maxillary nerve (V₂)

Mandibular nerve (V₃)

b

Anatomical location	Injury	Management
Cornea	Corneal rupture	Suturing if unstable; if stable, eye shield and close follow-up
	Corneal abrasion	Antibiotic eye ointment (chloramphenicol twice a day)
Anterior chamber	Hyphaema	Corticosteroid (dexamethasone four times a day); dilate (cyclopentolate twice a day); monitor for intraocular pressure daily until resolved, with strict bed rest
Iris	Traumatic mydriasis	No treatment
Lens	Cataract	Cataract extraction and artificial lens insertion
	Phacodonesis	If lens fibres are unstable this may require removal with placement of a more anterior artificial lens
Vitreous	Vitreous haemorrhage	Observe and monitor with ultrasound for signs of retinal detachment
Retina	Commotio retinae	No treatment but careful monitoring
	Retinal detachment/dialysis/tears	Vitreoretinal surgical input
	Choroidal rupture	If complete rupture, may require operation for primary repair; otherwise, observation
Optic nerve	Traumatic optic neuropathy	High-dose intravenous corticosteroid (1 g methylprednisolone daily for 3 days)
Orbit	Orbital floor fracture	Requires maxillofacial input with potential treatment by repair and plating

Table 15.3 Blunt injuries to the eye and orbit and subsequent management

Investigations

Investigations should include a radiograph of the orbit and face followed by CT scanning of the orbits. In addition, there should be ultrasound scanning of the globe if the view of the retina is unclear.

Management

Management varies widely according to the abnormalities found (**Table 15.3**).

Prognosis

Patients with central retinal or optic nerve pathology tend to do very poorly. A RAPD is a poor prognostic indicator.

Index

Note: Page numbers in **bold** or *italic* refer to tables or figures respectively.